CARNIVORE
The Manual

Compact Edition

By

Duncan Smart

*A Manifesto for
the Metabolic Rebellion*

Published by Ancestral Living Press

United Kingdom 2025

CARNIVORE: THE MANUAL

This book is a work of creative nonfiction. It blends metabolic science, ancestral memory, metaphor, and personal reflection. All scientific references are based on real evidence. Any symbolic or fictionalized content is used to illuminate, not obscure, the truth. Resemblance to real persons, living or undead, is often intentional.

This book includes satire, metaphor, and critical commentary protected under the principles of free expression and fair use. Any critique of individuals, corporations, government bodies, or institutions is intended as commentary on systems and ideologies, not as defamation or personal accusation. Medical and nutritional information is provided for educational purposes only and is not intended as a substitute for professional advice.

The author and publisher disclaim responsibility for any adverse effects resulting from the use or application of information contained in this book. Readers are encouraged to consult qualified professionals regarding health, diet, and medical decisions.

ISBN: 978-1-0682937-3-3

Distributed via Kindle, Draft2Digital, and other platforms

First Edition

Published in the United Kingdom. 2025

For more information:
www.carnivore-guide.com

To my father, Julian

The first to place flesh in my hands,
who weaned me on the wild
and taught me the
sacredness of the kill.

For Jacob, Harvey,
and Tabitha

You are the fire that forged me.

Jacob and Harvey,
you made me a father,
sharp as flint
and fierce in love.

Tabitha, my daughter,
you softened the steel
and made me whole.

Contents

Author's Note

This book carries the same heart, chapters, and message as *Blood & Bone: The Vampire's Guide to Carnivore Living*. The call to remember what you are is unchanged.

The original used the vampire as a metaphor for metabolic sovereignty, instinct, and ancestral truth. He was not chosen for drama, but for memory. He remembers what we have forgotten - how to be strong, untamed, and purposeful. How to refuse the feedlot and return to the fire.

Yet many never opened it. Some assumed it was fiction. Others were put off by the symbol before they could grasp the science. That's why this edition exists. The message is the same. But the package is simpler, sharper - a more direct path to the truth for those who need it.

Do not mistake this for a retreat. The vampire's voice remains where it matters. Because metaphor isn't decoration... it's delivery. A mythical figure can speak with a clarity that cuts through cultural noise. He doesn't flinch, apologize, or soften the truth.

And that is the precise, unflinching voice this truth requires.

Duncan Smart

<u>Prologue</u>

The Red Pill and the Raw Cut

In the beginning, there was blood, flesh and bone

You were told food is fuel. That blood is dirty. That hunger should be numbed, and cravings tamed.

They taught you to revile meat. To microwave convenience. To flatten instinct into guideline. You were fed sugar, seed oils, and softness. Histories without hunger. Oils without origin. You were domesticated.

But there's a part of you that remembers. It stirs in silence. In the crack of bone. In the scent of seared flesh. In the whisper of something older than farms in your veins.

It's the part that doesn't want to count calories. It wants to hunt. It doesn't want to moderate. It wants to devour. It sees the predator in the mirror and feels the flicker of fangs. I speak to that part.

This book is for the predator within.

You take the blue pill, the story ends. You wake up in your bed and believe whatever you want to believe. You take the red pill, you stay in Wonderland, and I show you how deep the rabbit hole goes.

Forget the rabbit. We're going deeper. Past nutrition science. Past macros. Past meal plans.

We're heading into myth, into predator and prey, into vampire and beast, Into the ancient stories where your hunger finds its true name and lineage. Because the domesticated mind fears science. But the awakened soul speaks myth.

Because food isn't just fuel. It's ritual. It's identity. It's rebellion. Vampires don't age. They don't get sick. And they damn sure don't eat cornflakes.

The vampire is not the villain. He is the awakened one who looked at a world sick on sugar and grain, smelled the rot beneath the perfume, and whispered: "This food is the lie. I choose blood. I choose strength."

He feeds with purpose. He fasts with intention. He does not ask permission. He eats like a god, not a slave. He is me. And he might be you, if you're willing.

Forget dirty blood. Forget numbed hunger. Forget the lie that called food "fuel."

This is your red pill. This is meat, myth, and blood. This is carnivore, resurrected as a vampire's manifesto.

Let's see how deep it goes

<u>Chapter 1</u>

Myths We've Been Fed

The deepest wound is not hunger. It is the lie that you were told that made you forget what you are.

You remember the moment. You opened the fridge, looked around, and thought: None of this feels right.

Maybe it was after your tenth low-fat Greek yogurt. Maybe it was watching someone microwave a plastic tray of beige while claiming "health." Maybe it was just a quiet instinct. A whisper in your blood: This isn't food.

You were inside the simulation and didn't know it.

In *The Matrix*, Neo stares at a steak. Juicy. Sizzling. Irresistible. But it's not real. It's code. An illusion built to sedate. Meanwhile, outside the simulation? Slop. Grayness. Bland sustenance. "I know this steak doesn't exist. I know that when I put it in my mouth, the Matrix is telling my brain that it is juicy and delicious… ignorance is bliss."

That's the modern food system. Hyper-palatable. Highly addictive. Carefully engineered to numb you while keeping you obedient.

Food that feeds no instinct. Calories that cost your clarity. A thousand options, none of which satisfy.

The Simulation Is Real

Supermarkets glow under cold LED light, filled with fake choices and fluorescent distractions. Cereal aisles thirty feet long. Plant-based meat engineered by software developers. Fruit flown from six time zones away, sugared to perfection, wrapped in plastic.

The Matrix isn't science fiction. It's your kitchen. Your school cafeteria. Your doctor's "heart-healthy" pamphlet.

You Were Designed to Devour

We didn't evolve eating this way. No tribe ever gathered around a microwave. No elder ever taught his sons how to track lentils.

We hunted. We fasted. We feasted. We tore muscle from bone and drank the blood warm.

Your DNA hasn't forgotten. It remembers the taste of marrow. The reverence of fire. The sound of fat hissing on stone.

You don't need a new diet. You need to unplug. You need to remember what food was, before it was branded, boxed, and blessed by influencers. You need to take the red pill and taste the raw cut.

Myth #1: Cholesterol Is The Enemy

The body produces 75% of its own cholesterol. Why? Because cholesterol is essential: to hormones, brain function, cell membranes, and healing. It's not the enemy. It's the scaffolding of life[1].

The war on cholesterol began with Ancel Keys and his infamous Seven Countries Study. Except it wasn't seven countries. It was twenty-two. He cherry-picked the ones that fit his narrative. Correlation dressed up as causation[2].

The result? Decades of low-fat guidelines, statin prescriptions, and a tidal wave of metabolic dysfunction. Heart disease didn't decline. It exploded[3].

Myth #2: Saturated Fat Will Kill You

Your ancestors ate saturated fat from wild game, bone marrow, and organ meat. They didn't die of heart attacks. They died when predators ripped their throats out.

Modern humans die differently. From insulin resistance. From inflammation caused by seed oils, ultra-processed carbs, and constant grazing. Not from a ribeye.

The saturated fat fear was never about health. It was about marketing: selling margarine, low-fat garbage, and sugar-laced "alternatives."

Myth #3: You Need A Balanced Diet

A 'balanced' diet. A little bit of everything. Moderation. Variety. That's not nutrition. That's surrender to the system's demands.

No predator eats a balanced diet. A lion doesn't nibble on berries to keep things colorful. A wolf doesn't count macros.

Yes, humans are omnivores. But adaptation doesn't equal optimization. You don't need balance. You need species-appropriate nutrition. That means meat, fat, and maybe salt. It means simplicity, not variety for variety's sake.

'Balanced' is code for, 'Keep eating the system's products.'

Myth #4: You Should Eat Often

Breakfast. Snack. Lunch. Snack. Dinner. Snack. Six times a day to "boost your metabolism."

Wrong. Every time you eat, insulin spikes. Every spike is a storage signal: store fat, don't burn it. Constant feeding trains your body to expect sugar. It cripples your ability to access fat stores and metabolic flexibility.

Your body was never designed for constant feeding. You evolved too fast. To wait. To hunt. Fasting isn't extreme; it's a default.

These lies weren't just mistakes. They were profitable errors. They fed industries. They created customers. They weakened predators and fattened prey.

And now you're waking up to it.

Myth #5: Breakfast Is The Most Important Meal Of The Day

Who told you that? Your mom? Your teacher? Your doctor? Try Kellogg's. The same Kellogg's that sold sugar-coated flakes to generations of sleepy-eyed children. The same Kellogg's that funded ad campaigns, "studies," and public-school programs. The same Kellogg's that turned a marketing slogan into a global gospel: "Breakfast is the most important meal of the day."

It didn't come from science. It came from John Harvey Kellogg, a Seventh-day Adventist who believed sexual urges were evil and that bland food, especially cereal, could suppress them[4].

Yes, really. The modern breakfast cereal industry was born not from nutritional wisdom, but from a desire to curb masturbation. And now we wake up and eat cornflakes and Pop-Tarts like we're in a sanitarium. Your body doesn't want cereal. It wants silence. It wants movement. It wants clarity.

Hunger in the morning isn't a deficiency; it's detox. It's a clearing of cellular waste. It's your body resetting.

But Kellogg's couldn't profit off your fasted clarity. They couldn't sell you a box of "don't eat." So they engineered a meal, then convinced you it was a need.

It wasn't. You don't need breakfast. You need freedom from habits you never chose, and hunger signals hijacked by sugar and starch.

Myth #6: Seed Oils Are "Heart-Healthy"

Canola. Soybean. Sunflower. Corn. Cottonseed. They call them 'vegetable oils,' but not even one comes from a vegetable.

These are industrial seed oils, born in factories, extracted with chemicals, and refined with bleach. They were never food. They were machine lubricants in the early 20th century before clever marketing put them on your plate[5].

What they really are: PUFAs - polyunsaturated fatty acids. Sounds like science. Sounds harmless. But they're molecularly unstable. They oxidize fast. They inflame your tissues. And once inside you, they hang around for months, embedded in your fat cells like metabolic landmines.

You were designed to burn saturated fat. Animal fat. Tallow. Suet. Butter. Not the sludgy runoff of chemically abused crops.

But seed oil was cheap, shelf-stable, highly profitable.

So Big Food made a deal with Big Medicine: Push PUFAs. Demonize meat fat. Manufacture a generation of soft, inflamed, compliant citizens. And it worked.

Obesity soared. Fertility dropped. Depression and autoimmune diseases exploded. And everyone kept eating like it was normal. But it wasn't normal. It was sabotage disguised as food.

Myth #7: The Food Pyramid Is A Nutritional Blueprint

And after they corrupted your fats, they came for your entire plate. It looked so official. So clean. So scientific. A neat little triangle, printed on school posters and cereal boxes. At the bottom: 6–11 servings of bread, rice, cereal, and pasta. At the top: meat and fat. Use sparingly.

You were told this was how to be healthy. But what it really was? A dietary manifesto designed by politicians, not scientists.

The original USDA food pyramid wasn't based on human biology. It was built to protect the grain industry. To subsidize surplus wheat and corn. To make sure Americans kept eating what America produced the most of: cheap carbohydrates[6].

Meat was expensive. Fat wasn't shelf stable. But grain? You could process it, box it, brand it, and sell it to everyone from toddlers to pensioners.

So, they stacked the base of the pyramid with poison and told us it was the foundation of life.

The result? Obesity rates tripled. Type 2 diabetes became a rite of passage. Children got fat on Pop-Tarts and 'whole grains.' And somehow… meat became the enemy.

You weren't nourished. You were domesticated. The pyramid didn't feed your strength. It fed your compliance.

No predator builds a pyramid out of wheat. No vampire eats six slices of bread and calls it survival. And your ancestors didn't starve through winters to be told pasta is a superfood.

You were born to eat from the top of the food chain: meat, marrow, blood, and fat. Not from the bottom rung of a corporate food ladder.

It's time to flip the pyramid. Burn it, even. And build a plate based on instinct, not industry.

Myth #8: Plant-Based Is Better For You, And The Planet

It's clean. It's kind. It's green. Or so they tell you. "Plant-based" is the marketing Trojan horse of the century. Wrapped in moral superiority, packed with synthetic imitations, and rolled straight into your conscience.

But what's inside? Ultra-processed soy sludge. Factory-made 'meat' alternatives engineered by software developers. Seed oils, gums, starches, and synthetic vitamins - all trying to mimic what meat already is.

You're not saving the planet. You're outsourcing your health to Nestlé, Unilever, and Beyond Meat's board of investors.

And plants? Plants aren't passive. They don't want to be eaten. They fight back with oxalates, lectins, saponins, and phytoestrogens. Chemical signals that challenge digestion[7]. They hijack your hormones. Wreck your gut lining. Pretend it's 'fiber.'

Cows don't need ingredient labels. But your oat milk does. A lion doesn't consult a nutritionist. Your soy burger requires a PhD in chemistry.

You were told meat is cruel. But monocropping fields to death with glyphosate and diesel isn't? Killing billions of insects, rodents, and soil microbes for tofu is peaceful?

The vampire doesn't graze. He doesn't sip pea milk under LED lights. He takes what he needs, with instinct, precision, and blood-soaked truth. So should you.

Myth #9: It's Just About Calories In vs. Calories Out

Let's break this illusion. That your body is a simple furnace. That weight loss is just math. That if you 'burn more than you eat,' you'll get lean.

DUNCAN SMART

Wrong. You are not a calculator. You are a hormonal symphony, not a spreadsheet.

Calories don't account for: Insulin levels: Leptin resistance; Ghrelin signaling; The thermic effect of food; The quality and bioavailability of nutrients[8]

100 calories of steak is not 100 calories of cereal. One nourishes, satiates, and builds. The other spikes insulin and leaves you hungrier than before.

Calorie counting is a cage. It turns you into a spreadsheet, not a predator. The carnivore doesn't count calories. He eats until the kill is gone. Then fasts. Then hunts again.

That's the cycle. Feast and fast. Not count and nibble.

Myth #10: You Need Fiber To Poop, Detox, And Thrive

You've been told that fiber is a broom. That it 'scrubs' your intestines clean. That it keeps you 'regular.' That it feeds your gut bugs and prevents cancer. And without it? Constipation. Toxicity. Certain death by irregularity. The truth? Fiber is overhyped plant residue your body never asked for.

Let's get primal. Your ancestors weren't waking up to overnight oats and chia pudding. They weren't crunching kale and beans to make sure they hit their 'recommended daily allowance.' They were eating animals. Nose to tail.

Organs, meat, collagen, marrow. And they weren't constipated - they were metabolically unchained.

Many people who eliminate fiber report: less bloating; more efficient digestion; cleaner, easier bowel movements[9].

Why? Because fiber can irritate the gut. Especially soluble and fermentable fibers, which feed the wrong microbes and can lead to: Gas and bloating; IBS symptoms; Constipation or diarrhea (yes, both).

Fiber doesn't 'clean' you - it often inflames you. And detox? That's handled by your liver and kidneys, not a spoonful of flaxseed[10].

Even observational studies linking fiber to reduced cancer risk often show weak or conflicting results. These are easily confounded by other dietary and lifestyle factors[11].

Yes, some individuals tolerate fiber well. But for many, cutting it unleashes true digestive sovereignty.

You don't need fiber. You need bioavailable nutrition, digestive rest, and a species-appropriate diet. A lion doesn't snack on roughage. A vampire doesn't chew kale. And you? You don't need fibrous filler. You need meat. Fat. Blood. Instinct.

Myth #11: You're Getting Enough Vitamin D

They tell you to avoid the sun. Lather up with SPF 50. Stay in the shade. Live like a vampire, they say - ironically, without the strength, hunger, or instinct. Then they hand you a bottle of vitamin D pills, pat you on the head, and send you back inside.

But here's the truth. Vitamin D isn't just a vitamin. It's a hormone. A master signal. A primal switch[12]. And it doesn't come in a soft gel. It comes from the sun hitting your skin, triggering a biochemical cascade that no supplement can truly replicate[13].

Nearly 1 billion people worldwide are deficient[14]. And deficiency isn't just about weak bones. It's tied to: Depression; Anxiety; Insulin resistance; Immune dysfunction; Cancer; Infertility; Fatigue; Brain fog; Hormonal collapse.

Why? Because modern life domesticates you. You're trapped indoors. Under fluorescent lights. Behind screens. You wake in the dark. You train in gyms. You eat under artificial bulbs. You live like a lab rat. And you wonder why you feel half-alive.

Your ancestors didn't supplement vitamin D. They chased it. They lived under it. Hunted in it. Bled in it.

The vampire myth flips here. Unlike the bloodless modern human, the vampire avoids the sun because it would reveal him. But you? You've been tricked into fearing the very thing that brings you to life. That's the real lie. We've become indoor creatures. Subdued. Sedated. Shadow-fed. When what we need is to stand in the light, bare-skinned, meat-fed, and wild.

They told you to fear the sun. They told you to fear cholesterol. But they never told you this. Vitamin D needs cholesterol to move. It's not just about making it in the skin. It's about transporting it, delivering it to tissues, activating it into its potent form.

And for that? You need the same thing they told you to cut out: fat. Specifically, LDL particles. The same ones that carry cholesterol also transport vitamin D: From the skin to the liver (calcifediol) Then to the kidneys (calcitriol), the active form your body actually uses[15]

No cholesterol? No transport. No activation. No vitamin D, no immune regulation, no testosterone, no bone health, no brain clarity.

So, when they told you to eat low-fat cereal, avoid red meat, and fear egg yolks? They didn't just rob your hormones. They disarmed your sunlight.

This is why the carnivore lifestyle resurrects health at the cellular level. It brings back cholesterol-rich animal fat, the bloodstream's FedEx system for fat-soluble vitamins like D, A, E, and K2.

You don't need fortified cereal. You need sunlight and steak. You don't need a supplement. You need blood, bone, and ancestral fire.

Myth #12: You Need 8 Glasses Of Water a Day

Let's be blunt. The '8-glasses-a-day' rule is arbitrary nonsense. It has no scientific basis. None. It came from a misinterpretation of a 1945 report. The original document said adults require about 2.5 liters of water daily... and then added: "Most of this is contained in food."[6] Guess which part everyone ignored?

So now we carry emotional support water bottles and sip all day like dehydrated lab rats, peeing out sodium, potassium, and magnesium with every over-hydrated bathroom trip. True hydration isn't about flooding your kidneys. It's about electrolyte balance.

And here's where the carnivore flips the script. Animal foods, especially red meat, bone broth, and salt. Provide the minerals you need to stay hydrated at a cellular level: Sodium (from salt); Potassium (from meat); Magnesium (from bone marrow and organ meats)[17].

Drink when you're thirsty. Add salt when needed. Don't micromanage nature. Your body is a primal feedback loop, not a spreadsheet.

And vampires? They're not sipping lemon water with chia seeds. They hydrate with blood: iron-rich, mineral-charged, ancestral fluid.

Hydration is about what you absorb, not how much you drink. It's about holding the water you do take in, not just flushing it out because you're obeying a number on a blog.

Myth #13: Saturated Fat Clogs Your Arteries

This one didn't just mislead people. It buried them. It sent generations into statin regimens, low-fat diets, and 'heart healthy' margarines. It stripped butter from their tables. It replaced tallow with soybean sludge. It told us that animal fat causes heart disease. And the world got sicker. Softer. Sadder.

But here's what they never told you: Your brain is 60% fat; Your hormones are built from cholesterol; Your cell membranes run on saturated fat. You're not just designed to tolerate it. You're built by it.

The theory that saturated fat causes heart disease has never been proven. Ever. The largest and most recent meta-analyses show no link between saturated fat intake and heart disease[18].

But here is what correlates: Refined carbs; Seed oils; Insulin resistance; Chronic inflammation[19]. You know - the very things people were told to eat instead of fat.

The rise of heart disease didn't happen before saturated fat was demonized. It happened after. And when you eat ancestral fats, tallow, suet, egg yolks, butter: You're not clogging pipes. You're rebuilding tissue. You're restoring hormonal balance. You're fueling the primal machinery of your body like it was meant to run.

The carnivore doesn't fear fat. He thrives on it. Dense, powerful, animal energy. The enemy wasn't on your plate. It was in your shopping cart. Your breakfast cereal. The food pyramid on your fridge.

Myth #14: Salt Raises Blood Pressure And Damages Your Heart

And while they robbed your fat, they came for your minerals next. They told you salt raises blood pressure. That it stresses your heart. That it should be avoided, restricted, swapped for low-sodium soups and salt-free snacks.

And the result? People walking around hyponatremic, sluggish, dizzy, insulin-resistant, and craving carbs. Because salt isn't a threat. Salt is primal electricity.

Your body is literally powered by sodium-potassium gradients. Every nerve impulse. Every muscle contraction. Every heartbeat - driven by electrolytes[20].

Cut your sodium too low and you don't just feel tired. You short-circuit. And guess what? When you go low-carb, when you return to the predator's fuel system, you lose water and sodium through the kidneys. That's why many carnivores and keto athletes feel off when they first start. They're still afraid of salt.

You don't need less salt. You need the right kind. Unprocessed. Mineral-rich. Unapologetically primal. Sea salt. Rock salt. Celtic salt. Not that iodized powder in the blue container, labelled as table salt, that tastes like chemical residue.

Let's talk history. Salt built empires. Roman soldiers were paid in salt - their 'salary.' Wars were fought over salt routes. Entire cities rose around salt mines and salt licks. Why? Because every living creature needs it. It preserves. It energizes. It nourishes.

But today? They'll warn you about salt while selling sports drinks full of sugar and synthetic chemicals. The vampire doesn't fear salt. He craves minerals. He knows the body's language: blood, water, salt, fat, fire.

Let the herd drink distilled sadness and count milligrams. You? You salt your meat. You salt your sweat. You salt your soul. Because without salt, the blood doesn't flow right.

Myth #15: Meat Takes Days To Digest And Rots in Your Colon

It's whispered in wellness circles: "Meat just sits in your gut. It rots. It's unnatural."

False. Meat leaves the stomach within 2–4 hours and is fully digested in the small intestine. Quickly. Thanks to potent stomach acid and enzymes, using bioavailable nutrients with near-total absorption[21].

It's kale, beans, and whole grains that bloat, gas, and ferment their way through your gut for days - while meat is long gone and assimilated. The vampire doesn't rot from meat. He runs on it… and so do you!

Myth #16: Eating Meat Is Immoral

Modern moral nutrition teaches: "To eat meat is to kill. To kill is cruel." But predators don't apologize for being predators.

Every bite you take costs life - plant or animal. Death isn't avoided in agriculture. It's industrialized and hidden behind fields of soy[22].

But ancestral meat-eating? It was direct. Sacred. Nose to tail. Honored. The vampire doesn't feast without reverence. He understands what is taken, and what is given. To eat meat with awareness is not immoral. It's primal. It's real.

Some argue over sentience and suffering. But the scale of death in industrial plant agriculture exceeds most imaginations. What matters isn't absence of death. It's presence of honor.

Myth #17: High Protein Will Damage Your Kidneys

This myth lingers like a bad gym rumor. There is no evidence that high-protein diets harm healthy kidneys. This idea came from renal patients and was wrongly applied to the general public[23].

Protein builds tissue. Protein fuels function. Protein heals. It doesn't harm.

Your ancestors didn't fear protein. They chased it.

Myth #18: Ketosis Causes Ketoacidosis

Ketosis and ketoacidosis are not the same. Nutritional ketosis is a natural metabolic state. Ketoacidosis is a life-threatening diabetic condition.

Conflating the two is like comparing a candle to a wildfire. Ketosis fuels the brain, preserves muscle, and burns fat cleanly[24]. It's how you were designed to survive famine. Even infants are in ketosis while breastfeeding[25].

Ketosis isn't dangerous. It's ancestral code.

Myth #19: Fasting Burns Muscle and Slows Your Metabolism

You've been told: "skip a meal and you'll waste away".

Wrong! Fasting increases growth hormone, improves insulin sensitivity, and activates autophagy. That's cellular recycling and regeneration[26].

You don't lose muscle by skipping meals. You lose it by eating garbage. The vampire doesn't graze. He waits. He sharpens. Then he feeds.

Myth #20: Carbohydrates Are Essential For Survival

There is no such thing as an essential carbohydrate. The body can make all the glucose it needs from protein and fat via gluconeogenesis[27].

Tribal carnivores like the Inuit, Maasai, and Chukotka ate near-zero carbs for generations.

Carbs aren't evil. But they aren't required. They're a tool. And for many… a trap.

Chapter 2

Dracula Doesn't Do Carbs

How hunger became a messenger, not a threat.

No vampire ever counted macros. His ledger is written in blood, not bread.

The modern world tracks calories as if the body were an accountant, balancing spreadsheets of sins and rewards. But Dracula doesn't snack. He doesn't sip. He waits. And when the time comes, he feeds.

Fasting isn't starvation. It's restraint. The pause before the pounce. A return to metabolic memory. In the silence between meals, the body doesn't wither... it awakens. Ketones replace glucose. Alertness sharpens. Inflammation recedes. Mitochondria light their fires again.

This chapter is not about suffering. It's about timing. It's about what happens when we honor the hunger, rather than fear it.

Because Dracula doesn't do carbs. Not because he's afraid, but because sugar is the softness of death. He avoids it like he'd avoid a vegan barbecue.

Fasting Is Older Than Fire

Fasting is not a bio hack. It's not a trend. It's a return.

Long before the invention of agriculture, or ovens, or even flint, fasting was a default state. The kill was never guaranteed. The feast followed the find. And when winter came, or the hunt failed, or the sun moved away, hunger was the test we passed by remembering who we were.

The Inuit of the north fasted through storms. The Maasai walked days to graze their cattle. The Himba mothers nursed children without snacking on almonds or protein bars. Hunger wasn't feared. It was faced.

Even plants fast. Deciduous trees fast through winter, diverting energy to roots. Dormant seeds wait decades for rain.

Life uses pause as preparation. You don't need constant fuel. You need to remember the fire inside you.

Blood & Ketones: The Science of Undead Energy

Dracula feasts on blood: nature's perfect fuel. Fat-adapted, mineral-rich, devoid of glucose's lie. The body, too, has a backup. When deprived of sugar, it turns inward, not in desperation but in design.

Fasting activates AMPK and sirtuins, the guardians of cellular repair[1]. Autophagy clears out damaged components[2]. Ghrelin, the so-called "hunger hormone," increases not just appetite, but alertness and growth hormone[3]. Fasting may even regenerate immune cells[4] and reduce inflammatory cytokines[5].

Ketones rise. Insulin drops. Clarity returns. And with it, an older kind of hunger... the kind that hunted.

Fructose is liver poison[6]. Glucose is cellular rust[7]. Excess sugar glycates your arteries into stained glass windows of decay: a cathedral to entropy[8].

Ketones calm neural storms for many, ignite fire for some. Your biology writes the script. They fuel the brain cleanly, reducing oxidative stress[9] and increasing GABA, the neurotransmitter of calm[10]. They may protect against Alzheimer's[11], stabilize mood, and even suppress certain cancers[12].

They are the vampire's metabolic fangs. The vampire doesn't sip nectar between meals. He doesn't graze. He burns clean.

In 1963, physiologist Philip Randle discovered a biochemical rivalry between fuels. Glucose and fat don't like to share. This Randall Cycle[28] adds scientific teeth to the vampire's discipline.

When glucose floods the system, it shuts the gate on fat oxidation. When insulin is low and fat is high, the reverse happens: sugar gets sidelined. But eat both together, and you jam the gears. The cell stalls. Metabolic flexibility disappears.

This is why predators don't snack on carbohydrates between kills. And why Dracula never sweetens his blood. Fat is fire. Carbs are fog. Together, they don't feed. You burn neither. You bloat.

Fasting as Initiation

In tribal cultures, fasting is more than metabolic. It's mythic. Vision quests, Sun Dances, and rites of passage often begin with hunger. Because hunger changes perception. It removes the veil of satiety and reveals the self beneath the mask.

The Menominee fasted alone in the forest until the spirits gave them a vision[13]. The Crow warriors danced for days without food or water, waiting for dreams to come[14]. A 2019 study of the Sioux Sun Dance showed fasting-induced cortisol shifts and ketone production that mirrored modern metabolic benefits[15].

These rites belong to cultures far older and wiser than ours, but the hunger they reveal lives in us all.

The body doesn't lie. It remembers. Fasting returns us to that ancestral conversation.

Your hunger is not a threat. It is a messenger.

Modern Methods: How to Fast

You don't need to dance for four days. You just need to wait.

Here are three accessible methods:

1. **OMAD (One Meal A Day):** Consume all calories within a 1-2 hour window. Excellent for simplicity, insulin sensitivity, and fat adaptation. One meal per day, ideally timed 3-4 hours before sleep to align with circadian repair, if well tolerated[16].

2. **Circadian Fasting (Time-Restricted Eating):** Eat within a 6-8 hour window, ideally during daylight hours[17]. Aligns with melatonin, cortisol, and insulin rhythms. Modern humans are not nocturnal predators. Align eating with sunlight, unless you've traded your soul for immortality.

3. **Extended Fasts (24–72 hours):** A deeper reset. Promotes autophagy, insulin sensitivity, and mental clarity[18]. Best practiced 1-2 times per month. Only for metabolically adapted individuals. Responses vary across individuals, especially with hormonal cycles, stress, or stage of life. Consult a physician if pregnant, nursing, diabetic, or unwell.

Some feel the fire fast. Others must pass through fog. Temporary fatigue or "keto flu" is common. Your body is remembering.

Breaking the Fast: Ritual Matters

Don't sprint into the feast. Start with broth rich in natural salt. Let minerals awaken your cells first. Then choose fat-first foods: eggs, liver, steak, salmon, marrow. Prioritize digestibility and nutrients. Avoid nuts, fiber bombs, or sugar that could shock the gut.

Prepare the meal with intention. Break the fast like a warrior.

The Hunger as Sacred Messenger

We've been taught to fear hunger. To suppress it with snacks. To medicate it with caffeine or carbs. To silence the signal.

But hunger, true hunger, is the return of instinct. It doesn't mean you're weak. It means your metabolism is working. It means the body is whispering: "I remember."

When you fast, mitochondria multiply[19]. Inflammation drops[20]. Stem cells awaken[21]. Ketones enter the bloodstream like ancient keys.

Your hunger is not a flaw. It's your first teacher.

The Vampire Within

Dracula terrifies not because he's monstrous, but because he mirrors the hunger we chain in our shadows. Jung called it the Shadow Archetype, the parts of ourselves we exile[22].

But the vampire didn't exile his hunger. He refined it. His hunger is disciplined, not desperate. He does not graze. He waits. He fasts with purpose. He feasts with precision. He doesn't sip smoothies between Zoom calls. He doesn't chew gum in traffic. He doesn't snack on oat bars made by people who fear butter. His metabolism is not a cage. It's a throne.

The modern eater tries to burn both fuels at once: glucose and fat, toast and butter, pasta and cream. But the cell was not made to dual fuel.

The vampire knows. He chooses the flame. He does not mix his macros like potions. He respects the fire. The Randall Cycle is written into his cells, just as it's written into yours. Burn clean or burn out.

Return to the Night

You were not born to graze. You were not designed to count. You were built to fast ... and to feast. You were born into cycles. Light and dark. Feast and famine. Not moderation. Motion.

This isn't about suffering. It's about re-entering the rhythm your ancestors danced. The one the vampire still remembers. When you fast, you remember what he never forgot.

Chapter 3

The Turning, Initiation Crises and Metabolic Transformation

The night she turned, her bones ached with ancestral fire. The sugar died first. Then came the hunger. Then the flame.

The Descent: Metabolic Death and Rebirth

You imagined clarity. Lightness. A manageable hunger. Instead: collapse. Shivers on the bathroom floor at 3 a.m. A metallic taste in your mouth. The conviction you've been poisoned.

This is not detox. This is resurrection. Your mitochondria have forgotten the fire. They speak only glucose. To relearn fat, they must burn the library of sugar. This is not withdrawal. It is metabolic arson.

Night One: Salt and the Ghost-Water Exodus

When carbohydrates vanish, insulin drops. Without insulin's message to retain sodium, your kidneys flush it out like a breached dam. Glycogen stores deplete, and for every gram lost, up to four grams of water follow. What drains from your tissues is not just fluid. It is memory. Structure. Fire.

Aldosterone, the hormone that helps retain sodium, lags several days behind. The result:

- Dizziness like standing at the edge of a cliff.
- Headaches boring into your skull.
- Cramps that seize muscles with ghostly fists.
- A sudden, irrational fear that you're dying.

As sodium drains, cortisol seizes the wheel. Norepinephrine wavers. What you feel isn't simple fatigue, it's a hormonal mutiny, a coup d'état staged by adrenal panic.

Salt, glycogen water, and potassium all fall. The scale may drop. But it is not fat you've lost. It is the ghost of sucrose evacuating your veins. Salt abandoned me first. I became a dried riverbed. Then the fire whispered: "Where water flees, blood returns."

Night Two: Gut Revolt and the Death of the Garden

Your gut becomes a battlefield. The bacteria that fed on fiber and sugar begin to die. In their final act of rebellion, they release lipopolysaccharides (LPS), endotoxins that seep through the gut lining, sparking an immune response that feels like an infection.

This is not infection. It is your immune system burning the last bridges to the garden world.

Prevotella and *Bifidobacterium* don't just starve; they attempt to persist. They shift neurotransmitter balances, screaming for sugar through chemical echoes. But their screams are the echoes of a collapsing empire.

Ninety percent of your serotonin isn't made in your brain. It's hoarded in your gut by grain-fed bacteria[12]. When they die, your mood plummets. This is not depression. It's liberation.

Your symptoms may include: Sulfurous diarrhea; Acid reflux; Dreams of bread, biscuits, and golden syrup; Waking in sheets soaked with sweat and shame

The bile surge is erratic. Gallbladders long silenced by low-fat dogma struggle to keep pace. Gut flora shift. Carbohydrate-loving *Firmicutes* begin to die. Fat-metabolizing *Bacteroidetes* and butyrate-producing *Roseburia* move in. The transition is violent.

"I vomited bile beneath the moon. My intestines twisted with the garden's dying lies. The microbes wailed: Feed us sugar. I answered: Burn."

The Girl Who Burned the Ghost

Eliza's fibromyalgia had convinced her that her bones were made of glass.

On Night Two, she dreamt of mucin-barren intestines, where starving bacteria had begun eating her gut lining. She awoke not to pain, but to a terrifying emptiness.

Her partner offered her toast, smeared with butter. She took it, held it, and threw it into the sink.

"Something ancient is stitching me back together," she whispered. "From the inside out."

Eliza's 'glass intestines' were real. Zonulin had spiked from microbial warfare, ripping apart the tight junctions of her gut lining. But *Roseburia* had begun to bloom. Butyrate flooded the colon wall. The emptiness she felt was not a void; it was the endotoxins retreating. A microbial ceasefire.

Night Three: The Flame Returns

This is when it changes. The sugar has gone. The microbes have stopped screaming. The bile flows cleaner. And in the liver, a signal stirs.

Beta-hydroxybutyrate (BHB) is not merely fuel. It silences NLRP3 inflammasomes, reprograms DNA by inhibiting histone deacetylases (HDACs), and stabilizes inflammatory responses[8].

Your mitochondria regain their ability to oxidize fat, a capacity suppressed by chronic glucose abundance[9].

Ketones flood the brain. They cross the blood-brain barrier and fuel neurons as an efficient alternative to glucose[9]. GABA, the calming neurotransmitter, rises.

Lactobacillus strains now colonizing your intestines convert glutamate into GABA, a microbial sedative for a brain long overstimulated by sugar. The silence you feel is bacteria rebuilding your nervous system.

You feel: Calm, but not tired; Sharp, but not anxious; Clear, but not euphoric. This is not high. It is alignment.

I tasted marrow. The fire knew my name. Hunger became a compass, not a cry for mercy.

The Science of the Turning

1. **Sodium Resurrection:** Around days 3 to 5, aldosterone rises. Blood volume stabilizes. Salt cravings roar. Honor them. Without sodium, norepinephrine cannot bind to its receptor[5]. Salt is the spark that reclaims alertness.
2. **Bile Reawakening:** Cholate transforms into deoxycholate. This secondary bile acid activates FXR and TGR5 receptors in the gut and liver, resetting fat metabolism and initiating toxin clearance[12]. The liver remembers its fangs.
3. **Microbial Coup:** Sugar-loving *Firmicutes* fall. Fat-metabolizing *Bacteroidetes* rise. *Roseburia*'s butyrate heals the gut lining[7]. Candida fungi, starved of glucose, collapse.
4. **Neurochemical Recalibration:** Gut-brain crosstalk re-establishes. Dopamine and serotonin no longer answer to sugar-fed captors[8]. The cravings fall silent not because you resisted, but because the enemy was exiled.

5. **Epigenetic Signal:** BHB doesn't just feed, it transforms. It activates genes long silenced by glucose abundance, turning back on the metabolic code written in your blood[8].

Ritual Tools for the Turning

1. **Salt the Wound:** 5g sodium, 1g potassium, 400mg magnesium daily. Use sea salt, not supplements alone. Bone broth is liquid resurrection[3].
2. **Sleep Like the Dead:** Darkness. Silence. No alarms. Cortisol regulation begins in REM.
3. **Eat Lean, Then Rise:** Start with leaner cuts. Let bile production build. Add fat with intention[2].
4. **Bitter Herbs at Dusk:** Dandelion root or artichoke extract before the evening meal. Bitters activate TGR5 and prepare the gallbladder for the night's kill.
5. **Move Like a Predator:** Walking aids lymph drainage and bile flow. Stretching tames cortisol. Do not "train through" the purge. Let the fire recalibrate.

You are not sick. You are turning. The fire hurts before it heals. The vampire bled, too

Chapter 4

You Are Not Cattle

The greatest cages are built of comfort, routine, and fear. Freedom isn't given. It's hunted, earned, and remembered.

The Trough or the Wild

You were not born with a tag in your ear, a feed schedule, or a lifetime pass to the trough. You were not made for confinement, for the dull routine of grazing, or the glazed stare of the herd. But modern life would have you believe otherwise.

Supermarkets herd you down fluorescent aisles. Nutritionists tell you to graze: six meals a day, endless snacks, eat what's easy, what's fortified, what's been processed to death and then "enriched" for your safety. You're measured, counted, weighed, and fed the same advice given to livestock: "Eat your grains. Drink your low-fat milk. Stay docile."

But you are not cattle. You are the apex descendant of a million generations of hunters: wolf, not sheep; predator, not prey. Beneath layers of comfort and compliance, that wildness is still there, waiting.

Domestication: The Great Betrayal

Domestication is the story modernity calls progress. But it is also the story of the wolf, caged until his fangs dull. Of the wild aurochs, ancestor of modern cattle, hunted to extinction and replaced with docile beasts. Of the human animal, trading danger and freedom for safety and control.

Your ancestors once roamed vast plains, tracking herds, outwitting lions, thriving on hunger and uncertainty. Now, most humans are penned - body and mind - by systems designed to extract obedience and suppress resistance.

Grain-Fed Dependence

Grain is the food of the captive. Every animal in the feedlot eats it, not by choice, but because it's cheap, abundant, and easy to store.

Grain is the keeper's choice: cheap to grow, easy to ration, perfect for softening the edge of a once-sharp species.

So it is with humans. The modern "balanced diet" is built on bread, cereal, pasta, rice - foods our ancestors never relied on. Foods that fill but don't fortify. That sedate but don't strengthen.

Grains spike insulin, store fat, inflame and dull. Meat ignites ketones, burn fat, repair and sharpen. The feedlot runs on glucose. The wild runs on blood.

The result? Sluggish minds, anxious hearts, bodies buried in fat. These are not the burdens of the wild. They are the burdens of the feedlot.[1]

While some traditional agrarian cultures, like the Kitavans and Okinawans, thrived on starchy staples, their resilience came from natural rhythms, not industrial sedation. The modern grain problem isn't just grain. It's grain plus sugar, seed oil, and submission.

Biology of the Domesticated Animal

Russian geneticist Dmitry Belyaev proved that breeding for tameness changes everything. Within generations, silver foxes lost their fear, but also their sharpness. Their coats changed. Their ears flopped. Their instincts faded.[2]

Humans show the same signs: flatter faces; smaller jaws; dulled aggression.[3] We were not born this way. We were bred this way.

The Fossil Record Speaks

Compare skeletons: Before agriculture: Tall. Robust. Strong jaws. Minimal tooth decay. After agriculture: Shorter. Weaker. More cavities. Signs of anemia, arthritis, insulin resistance.[4]

Why? Because we traded wild meat and fat for porridge, bread, and starvation dressed as feast.[5] Armelagos' 2014 update shows a 40% rise in skeletal lesions, and a 30% drop in stature in grain-based populations.[6]

Domestication as Metaphor: The Tamed Mind

Domestication doesn't end with bodies. It tames the mind. We're taught to suppress instinct, to follow "expert" advice, to silence hunger with snacks. We're programmed to obey algorithms and avoid discomfort.

Comfort numbs hunger, but it also numbs desire, clarity, and courage. Grazing doesn't just dull the body. It dulls the will. Comfort needn't be decay. It can be a pause. But without risk, it becomes rot.

But the vampire rejects this. He fasts. He waits. He feeds on his own terms. To remember hunger is to reclaim power.

The Tray and the Fence

He sat in a school cafeteria, a tray in front of him: a milk carton, a slice of spongy bread, a plastic cup of fruit cocktail. He didn't eat.

He pushed the tray away, milk carton toppling, fruit cocktail bleeding red syrup across the table. A teacher snapped: "Eat!"

He stood. The fence, though invisible, screamed behind him.

The Wild Versus the Captive

Tribal cultures have always understood captivity's cost.

The San (Southern Africa): San hunters fasted while tracking antelope to sharpen focus. When one man stole settler grain, elders warned: "Eat like the white man, and you will grow slow like his cattle."

The Inuit: They prized wild caribou and saw the penned as weak.[7] The Maasai: Raised on blood, milk, and meat, low in grains, high in power. Among the leanest, healthiest people recorded.[8]

The Tsimane (Bolivia): Live on wild meat, tubers, and constant movement. Despite chronic inflammation, they show almost no coronary artery disease.[9]

But wilderness is no utopia. It feeds the prepared, not the romantic. The wild requires reverence and readiness, lest it punish those who wander unarmed.

The Feast and the Fence

Imagine a tribal hunt. The morning silence, the sharpened spear, the painted faces, the fasted bodies humming with tension. The tribe surrounds the animal. It is not just food, it is spirit, risk, and ritual.

Now imagine a factory farm: A steel chute. A sedated animal. A man with a bolt gun on shift rotation. No prayer. No hunger. No story.

Modern humans eat in fluorescent silence. Lunch is scheduled, not earned. The body is trained to salivate at the sound of a bell, not the sight of a kill.

The sacred rhythm of scarcity and reward has become the shameful routine of grazing at noon.

The Deep Roots of Domestication

Ten thousand years ago, everything changed. Grain took over. Fields replaced herds. Wheat and barley became gods. The aurochs was penned. The hunter became the farmer. Control replaced chaos.[10]

Grain wasn't just calories. It was control. Storable. Taxable. Rationable. Kings built granaries before thrones. The first chains were woven from wheat.

Civilization and the Feedlot

The first cities were granaries. Grain allowed taxation and hierarchy. From Babylon to Rome, the pattern was the same, feed the masses, tame the masses.

Bread and sugar didn't just nourish empires. They pacified them.[11] Rome rotted from within on wheat-dole and lead-sweetened wine. We decay on seed oils and soda.

Even today, the most 'advanced' societies are the sickest.

Modern Rebels: Carnivore Athletes and Rewilders

The wild isn't just remembered. It's being reborn. Zach Bitter, endurance runner, thrives on zero carbs. Shawn Baker, 57-year-old ex-orthopedic surgeon, breaks rowing records. His bones remember what bran flakes forgot… density requires danger.

Amber O'Hearn, neuroscientist and mother, rewilded her family on meat and marrow. "Carnivory nourishes minds meant to roam."

The Nenets: Siberian children eat raw reindeer and frozen fat. No vitamins. No medicine. Just instinct, fire, and blood.[12] [13]

The Vampire Who Broke the Fence

Once, a vampire lived quietly among the herd. He fed gently, just enough to stay comfortable. But every night, as he wandered through the city, he felt a tug… something ancient, something wild.

One evening, he followed it. Past the neon. Beyond the fences. Into the dark woods at the city's edge. There, he met another of his kind, older, leaner, eyes burning with hunger and memory.

"Why do you linger among the herd?" the elder asked. "It's easy," said the young one. "I am never hungry." The elder smiled with ancient fangs. "Then you are already dying." "But I am safe," said the young vampire. "Safety is the fence," said the elder. "Comfort is the cage. Hunger is the fire."

And so, the younger tore the fence with his teeth, tasting rust, freedom, and centuries of stolen hunger. He felt his veins blaze. His hunger wasn't myth. It was mitochondrial. His blood ran ketones. His clarity returned.

For the first time in centuries, he was alive.

You Are Not Cattle

You are not cattle. You were not born to graze. You were not made to obey. Predator, not prey. Forged, not fed. You were built to fast and feast, To kill. To kneel only to the hunt. To thank the blood. To break the fence. To choose the wild. To remember.

How to Rewild Yourself

1. **Eat Like a Predator** Ditch grazing. Abandon grain. Feast on meat, fat, organs, eggs, then stop. Fast until true hunger returns. Liver weekly. Marrow as dessert.
2. **Move Like a Hunter** Walk. Sprint. Climb. Lift. Carry. Train outdoors. Mimic the persistence and explosiveness of ancestral hunters.
3. **Embrace Hunger** Let it sharpen your senses. Let it teach you to wait, focus, and act with intention.

4. **Fast with Intention** Try OMAD. Experiment with 24-hour fasts. Turn fasting into ritual. Reflect, walk, or train as you fast.

5. **Seek Wildness** Get cold. Get hot. Get dirty. Touch trees. Swim in rivers. Sleep outside. Let rain sting your skin. Let wind scour your domestication.

6. **Question the Feedlot** Who profits from your softness? Who benefits from your compliance? Reject their comfort, but not your conscience. Choose the unknown with eyes wide.

7. **Create Rituals** Make eating sacred. Make movement intentional. Use fire, song, or solitude. Ritual restores meaning.

8. **Connect to Ancestral Stories** Read them. Tell them. Live them. Howl their names: Aurochs. Steppe. Spear.

Chapter 5

The Original Diet Was Red

To eat flesh is to remember who we were - before agriculture, before empires, before sin.

Blood on the Grasslands

Picture it: the Pleistocene dawn, raw and golden. A lone hominin stands over the twitching body of a fallen beast. There's no fire, no seasoning, no polite separation of muscle groups. Just stone tools and a hunger deeper than the marrow being scooped from a cracked femur. This isn't a snack. It's survival. Transformation. Evolution in action.

The food pyramid never fed our evolution. The original diet wasn't balanced. It was iron-rich and fat-laced. It was forged in the furnace of need, carved into existence with obsidian edges. And it made us.

Long before fire kissed flesh, we were slicing into rib cages and sucking brain from skulls. Long before words, we had rituals. Long before empires, we had meat.

This chapter is about the red path: the ancient, sacred, and bloody route that shaped the predator behind the polite smile.

Bones, Stones, and Brains

The archaeological record doesn't lie. Fossils tell the story of our ascension through blood and bone. In places like Olduvai Gorge, cut marks on animal skeletons dating back 2.5 million years reveal early hominins scavenging and butchering long before fire was mastered[1].

These weren't fruitarians on a cheat day. These were meat-hungry minds learning to crack open femurs for marrow: the original brain food.

According to the "Expensive Tissue Hypothesis," human evolution involved a critical biological trade-off[2]. A high-energy brain meant something had to give, and that something was gut length. Plant-eaters need long, complex intestines. Meat-eaters? Short, efficient systems built for dense nutrition.

When our ancestors began prioritizing fat, offal, and protein, our guts shrank, and our skulls swelled.

Anthropologist Richard Wrangham traces this leap in brain size to the rise of Homo erectus, around 1.8 million years ago[3]. Meat wasn't a supplement. It was the fuel. And the shift wasn't about cooking yet. It was about cutting, cracking, and consuming.

Before Prometheus gave us fire, the flesh gave us fire of the mind.

And with every cracked bone and marrow-fed brain, the ritual began to form. Not just the ritual of the hunt, but the myth, the meaning, the memory. Meat didn't just feed the body. It fed the story.

Every advancement, toolmaking, language, social cooperation, sprang from the evolutionary surplus meat provided. We didn't climb the food chain by chewing cud. We sprinted up it with a bloodied jaw.

The Predator in the Mirror

Modern comforts mask our predatory blueprint.

We sweat like marathoners. Our glutes, those juicy slabs we now park in ergonomic chairs, evolved for endurance hunting[4]. Our shoulders are engineered for throwing, our eyes for depth perception, and our stomach acid. A biological weapon. Human gastric pH is among the most acidic in the animal kingdom, rivaling vultures[5].

That's not for digesting salad. That's for killing bacteria found in carrion and raw flesh. We are built, inside and out, for meat.

Even our brains reflect predation. Foresight. Tool use. Cooperation in the hunt. Empathy isn't just a moral trait. It evolved to enhance teamwork during the kill. We're apex predators with anxiety and Google Calendars.

And yes, this wasn't a solo performance by males with spears. In many hunter-gatherer societies, women participated in hunting persistence prey or coordinated complex scavenging. They were often the first to access nutrient-rich organs, like liver, and they passed on the knowledge of animal processing through generations. The red path was shared.

Among the Hadza of Tanzania, women hunt small game, craft traps, and actively participate in meat acquisition: a living echo of our deep ancestral pattern. In contrast, other cultures like the Inuit or Nivkh show a clearer division, with women specializing in meat preparation rather than large-game hunting. Yet even there, the spiritual stewardship of flesh remained communal.

Among the Agta of the Philippines, women actively hunt wild boar with spears, proving the predatory spirit crossed gender lines when the environment demanded it.

And yet we flinch at this truth. We shrink from it, distracted by quinoa and guilt. But the truth remains: we are predators, not by choice but by design.

Blood isn't violence. It's memory. The original nutrient. A whisper from the ancestors that says: this is who you are.

Symbolism of the Kill

To kill is to cross a threshold. Not just of morality, but of transformation. Ancient peoples knew this. That's why hunting rites are often initiation rites. The boy kills, and becomes something new. The man, or woman, who feeds the tribe is reborn in blood.

Meat has always carried more than calories. It carries power. Myth. Memory.

In tribal societies, the liver is sacred. The heart is honored. The animal's spirit is thanked. Modernity has sterilized this into shrink-wrapped oblivion. But the old rituals knew: to take a life is to confront death, and by doing so, to affirm your own.

Among the !Kung of the Kalahari, a hunter apologizes to the slain antelope before butchering it, whispering that the kill was necessary to feed his family. The Nootka whale hunters of the Pacific Northwest conduct elaborate ceremonies to honor the spirit of the whale before consumption. The sacred kill was never just about food. It was about relationship.

The vampire is merely the symbolic extension of this truth. He doesn't farm. He doesn't apologize. He feeds with purpose, with instinct, with ancient certainty. The vampire doesn't farm because he refuses the feast of glucose. He thrives on blood, not bread.

In many oral traditions, women didn't just prepare the meat. They carried its myth.

Blood is life. It always was. That's why it sits at the heart of myth, of religion, of story. The sacred and the savage drink from the same wound.

The Fall into Agriculture: Bread Over Bone

But this predatory design collided with a new world, one that traded marrow for millet, and instinct for obedience. Then came the seeds.

The Neolithic Revolution, often praised as the birth of civilization, was really the beginning of our decline[6]. We traded wild meat for monoculture. We planted wheat and harvested weakness.

Bones don't lie. Early agrarian humans were shorter, more disease-prone, and less robust than their hunter-gatherer ancestors[7]. Caries and cavities appear in skulls where once there were only perfect teeth gnashing sinew.

Yes, agriculture enabled population growth and urbanization, but at the cost of metabolic vitality and skeletal integrity. And it spread not only through submission, but also through necessity: stored grain could withstand climate volatility. It was the logic of famine prevention, not metabolic enhancement.

But over time, farming favored predictability. It rewarded routine. You don't need a strong back to sow barley. You need obedience. Civilization didn't rise from strength. It rose from compromise.

Even the Bible reflects this shift. Abel the shepherd is slain by Cain the farmer. Eden is lost not through rage, but through appetite - for the wrong food. Bread becomes the symbol of toil, of exile, of dependency.

The vampire never tills the soil. He feasts. He remembers.

Remembering the Red Path

To walk the red path is not to return to a fantasy of the past. It's to reclaim what was never truly lost. The predator, the hunter, the blood-lit soul of humanity still burns beneath the surface. Every steak, every fast, every primal decision is an invocation.

The carnivore lifestyle isn't extreme. It's ancient. It's ancestral. It's aligned. It doesn't just feed the body. It reawakens the spirit. It whispers to the mitochondria, "I remember." It says no to submission, and yes to sovereignty.

Yes, modern humans have evolved to digest more starch, with extra amylase genes added to the mix... but that's adaptation to availability, not allegiance. Our core design still favors density, not dilution.

Because the red path is not just where we came from. It's where we return, sharpened by modern strength and ancient instinct. And sometimes, returning means not eating at all. Because before there was a feast, there was a fast.

Eat like your cells remember. Feast like your ancestors never left.

Chapter 6

Blood, Brine, and Bone - Humanity's Evolution to Eat Meat

The body does not lie. It may forget, but it does not fabricate. In bone and gut, in acid and blood, the truth endures... we were born to kill.

The Forgotten Flesh

Somewhere between savannah and shoreline, between fire and flood, humanity was forged. Not as a gardener of Eden, but as a predator of blood and fat. Our biology remembers what culture tries to forget. We are not gentle grazers. We are not gatherers of kale and compliance. We are flesh-eaters, evolved through muscle and marrow, shaped by necessity, sharpened by death.

The modern diet, wrapped in plastic and denial, muzzles the predator's growl. Yet myths persist, and in them - lurking beneath garlic and gravestones - is the echo of our evolutionary truth.

This chapter reclaims that truth. Through the lens of anatomy, anthropology, and archetype, we uncover the unmistakable evidence: humans evolved to hunt, to eat meat, and to devour with the efficiency of a born predator. Even the controversial Aquatic Ape Hypothesis, often dismissed, offers insights into our early adaptations to fat, salt, and blood.

The Gut Speaks: Anatomy of a Hunter

A Gut Built for Absorption, Not Fermentation

The human digestive tract is an evolutionary blueprint, a schematic not of what we believe we should eat, but of what we were forged to consume.

Humans have a long small intestine (constituting roughly 56–67% of the total gut volume) and a short colon (about 17–23%)[1]. This is the inverse of what we see in herbivores, whose lengthy colons and large ceca are fermentation factories for plant matter.

Our vestigial cecum, a hollow pouch with minimal function, offers further evidence. It is a relic of herbivorous ancestry, now obsolete in the carnivore-leaning physiology of Homo sapiens[2].

While we retain some ancestral capacity for plant digestion - such as amylase enzymes for starch - our gut is optimized for nutrient-dense absorption from animal foods.

Stomach Acidity: Death by Digestion

Human stomachs operate at a remarkably low pH (~1.5), comparable to scavengers such as vultures[3]. This extreme acidity is not required for digesting plant foods but is crucial for denaturing proteins and killing pathogens in raw or aged meat. It is a predatory adaptation hidden in plain sight. High gastric acidity in humans is consistent with a dietary history involving the regular consumption of animal tissues.[3]

Shoreline Predators: The Aquatic Ape Revisited

Elaine Morgan's Aquatic Ape Hypothesis (AAH) challenged the prevailing savannah model by suggesting that key human traits evolved in a waterside environment. Though debated, the AAH's emphasis on shoreline predation aligns with fossil evidence of early human seafood consumption and coastal foraging adaptations.

Fossilized shell middens at Pinnacle Point (c. 164,000 years ago) reveal that early humans exploited marine resources long before agriculture. This suggests that salt, fat, and iodine shaped our brains as much as the hunt on land.

Traits of the Water-Forager

Morgan and others identified traits that may indicate semi-aquatic adaptation:

- Hairlessness: for streamlined swimming, as seen in aquatic mammals
- Subcutaneous Fat: for insulation and energy storage, found in marine carnivores

- Breath Control: essential for diving and, interestingly, a precondition for speech
- Bipedalism: useful in shallow water wading and fishing[4]

This was not a gentle swim through paradise. It was a hunt. The water was not for sipping; it was for stalking.

These adaptations hint not at a herbivorous forager, but at a coastal predator. A hominin capable of catching fish, cracking bones, and accessing dense sources of fat and protein.

Evolution on the Estuary

Coastal and estuarine environments offered predictable, high-calorie food sources:

- Shellfish, fish, sea mammals - the crack of shell, the slick salt of marrow
- Nutrient-dense foods high in DHA, iodine, B12, and heme iron, all critical for brain development[4]

Waterside habitats offered early hominins a rich, energy-dense menu... even without advanced hunting tools.[4] This perspective reframes our ancestors not as fruit-pickers, but as shoreline apex foragers, preying upon the sea's bounty with growing sophistication.

Just as the sea shaped our bodies, myth shaped our hunger. Eternalized in the vampire's thirst.

The Vampire Archetype

The vampire, long seen as a mythical aberration, instead mirrors our suppressed biological truth. A being of cold logic and raw appetite, driven by bloodlust because blood was once the ultimate ancestral food.

Blood is rich in Heme iron, a form far more bioavailable than that in plants. Plasma proteins, essential amino acids, and nutrients like zinc, selenium, and B12

Traditional carnivorous cultures such as the Maasai, Inuit, and Mongols regularly consumed blood, often raw or mixed with milk or meat[5].

In Maasai tradition, warriors drink blood mixed with milk from a living cow. This symbolizes strength, nourishment, and reverence. The cow is not slaughtered. Its blood is tapped and shared. This is no act of cruelty. It is a ritual of communion with life itself.

While blood was ritually prized, organs like liver and marrow offered similar nutrients with less microbial risk. Evidence of a sophisticated, risk-aware predator. The vampire's thirst is not metaphor. It is nutritional instinct made eternal.

Aversion to the Agricultural World

The vampire cannot stomach garlic, bread, or wine. It is burned by the Eucharist. These are not random folkloric tropes. They are symbols of agricultural civilization:

grain, grape, herb. The vampire is not just anti-Christian. It is anti-agriculture. It is a relic of the predator age, cast as a villain by the grain-fed masses.

"Lycaon, king of Arcadia, dared to serve Zeus human flesh. As punishment, he was transformed into a wolf - condemned to stalk the wild forever, feeding on blood and bone." - Ovid, Metamorphoses

Even in myth, those who feed on flesh are feared, exiled, and immortalized. The vampire's relentless focus mirrors the mental clarity of ketosis. A metabolic state our ancestors accessed through fasting and feasting.

The Brain-Gut Tradeoff

The Expensive Tissue Hypothesis holds that as the human brain expanded; the gut shrank. But this trade-off is only sustainable if the diet delivers dense, easily digested energy - animal fat and cooked meat[6].

Cooking meat reduces chewing time and increases calorie availability. It wasn't about taste. It was evolution. Meat fed the brain. The brain fed our rise. Cooking led to a reduction in gut size and an increase in brain volume - a shift impossible on raw plant diets.[6]

The Cognitive Kill

Hunting demands: Planning; Tool use; Language; Social cooperation. These cognitive leaps co-evolved with meat consumption. Our brains grew not because we foraged better, but because we hunted better[7]. We were built to strategize, stalk, and kill. Our intelligence is an outgrowth of the kill.

The Grain Rebellion: How Agriculture Softened the Predator

Agriculture changed the world, but it did not improve our biology. It prioritized calories over vitality, and volume over strength.

It wasn't progress. It was a compromise. The plough didn't feed strength. It fed numbers.

The Decline Begins

With grain came: Iron deficiency anemia; Tooth decay; Stunted growth; Micronutrient deficiencies[8]

These diseases of civilization are visible in Neolithic skeletons. The wildness of the predator was tamed by the yield of the plough.

The Myth of Progress

Civilization rewards docility, not hunger. It tells us not to eat meat, not to fast, not to kill.
And yet - our bodies remain built for it.

Like the vampire, we have been cast as monsters for remembering what we are.

The Flesh Remembers

We are the predator pretending to be prey. The vampire pretending to be vegan. The shoreline hunter trapped in a field of wheat.

You may deny the kill. But your cells remember. Your blood remembers. And when the hunger comes, it will not be for wheat. Feed the memory. Hunt the hunger. Reclaim the brine and bone.

Eat Like a Shoreline Predator

- Prioritize omega-3-rich seafood: fatty fish, shellfish, sea mammals if available
- Fast like tidal rhythms: periods of absence followed by feasting
- Salt like the sea: embrace natural sodium intake, crucial for cognition and cravings
- Eat nose-to-tail: marrow, blood, liver - ancestral foods of the apex forager
- Reject modern myths: grains, seed oils, sugar, and fear
- Honor the kill: with reverence, with ritual, with memory

Chapter 7

The Salt That Remembers - Fire, Flesh, and the Forgotten Mineral

Take it with a grain of salt, and you may remember the truth it carried.

You can live without sugar. You can survive without fiber, fruit, or greens. But without salt, you die.

Salt is not seasoning. It is substance. It is covenant. It is the crystallized whisper of oceans that once flooded our blood. It does not expire. It does not rot. It remembers.

The vampire knows this. He salts his liver with care. He salts his past. He does not cramp on the hunt. He does not forget the fire. He does not fall, twitching, with blue lips and hollow eyes, lost in the saltless fog that weakens prey. He is charged. He is clear. He is salted.

The Covenant of Crystals

In the temples of old, salt sealed the sacred. Jewish priests offered it with every burnt sacrifice: "You shall not let the salt of the covenant be lacking"[1]. In Christian baptismal rites, salt touched the infant's tongue before the water reached the crown. In Japanese sumo, salt purifies the ring before battle. In Slavic folktales, salt was more precious than gold - a gift of loyalty and of love.

Salt protected what mattered. It preserved flesh, blood, and memory. When humans began to bury their dead with grave goods, salt was among the earliest tokens. It stood against decay.

Roman soldiers were paid in salt, salarium, a root word that lives on in salary. A typical salarium could buy enough salt to preserve thirty pounds of flesh each month. Mongol herders packed salt-dried organs for long winter rides. African traders carried slabs of salt across the Sahara to exchange for gold. Venetian empires rose on salt monopolies. When they lost control of the salt trade to the Turks, their dominance crumbled[2].

From the pink veins of Himalayan salt mines to the Celtic coasts where brine was boiled in clay pots, salt was sought like treasure.

Salt built cities. Salt started wars. Salt preserved the dead and remembered the living. Salt is memory made mineral.

The Metabolism of a Predator

We are wired for salt. Every cell in the body requires sodium to fire.

The carnivore, like the vampire, must guard this mineral closely, especially in the absence of carbs. Glucose promotes sodium retention. But when you eat only meat and fat, your kidneys excrete sodium more readily, and salt must be replenished with intention.

On a low-carb or ketogenic diet, inadequate salt leads to:

- **Adrenal stress**: Without enough sodium, aldosterone surges to compensate, triggering fatigue, dizziness, and cravings[3]. Cortisol rises in parallel, mistaking low salt for starvation.
- **Brain fog and weakness**: The sodium-potassium pump, which powers cellular electrical activity, begins to sputter.
- **Muscle cramps**: Electrolyte misfires.
- **Low blood volume**: You lose water with glycogen, and sodium follows, resulting in light-headedness and headaches.

You are not dying. You are desalted. You are drained of memory, disconnected from biological rhythm.

Dr. Tim Noakes has written extensively on sodium needs in endurance athletes, especially those following low-carbohydrate regimens. He emphasizes that sodium restriction in such individuals can be not just unnecessary, but dangerous[4].

The vampire's clarity depends on sodium, and its elemental kin. Salt is not flavor. It is fire.

The Paleolithic Palate

What did ancient humans do before salt mines? Before packaged electrolytes? They followed blood.

Our ancestors consumed whole prey - blood, bone, organ, and all. Blood itself contains sodium. So does bone marrow. The kidneys and adrenals of hunted animals contain a spectrum of electrolytes. Some tribes even consumed earth salts and clay from natural licks, just like deer do[5]. In coastal areas, seawater and dried marine salts were consumed. In alpine regions, salt was mined from rock veins like the famed Hallstatt deposits of ancient Austria.

A liter of mammalian blood contains around 3 grams of sodium - enough to sustain a day's hunt[6]. But blood was only one part of the ancestral mineral code.

The Inuit drank blood and ate raw kidney. The Hadza drank bone marrow broth. The Maasai, famed for their strength and height, regularly consumed a mix of blood, milk, and meat: a combination that preserved hydration, electrolytes, and hyponatremia resistance.

In cold climates, when blood was drained and frozen meat relied on preservation, salt was traded or mined. In warm lands, it was harvested from tidal flats, evaporated in ceramic basins, or scraped from the edges of mineral springs.

Paleolithic sodium intake is estimated to have been far higher than the intakes now recommended by public health authorities[7]. And unlike today's imbalanced sodium-chloride loads, ancestral salt was often buffered with potassium-rich animal tissue and occasional ash residue, protecting against acid-base disruption and bone loss. Salt wasn't optional. It was instinctive. The vampire remembers.

The Salt Deception

The demonization of salt may be one of the greatest nutritional sleights of hand in history.

Public health campaigns told us that sodium raises blood pressure. But they ignored context - specifically the inflammatory and insulin-driven terrain in which salt becomes problematic.

In metabolically broken bodies, swollen with sugar, seed oils, and chronic stress, sodium can indeed exacerbate existing dysfunction. But it is not the cause.

A 2014 paper in *Open Heart* exposed the farce: "It is not salt but sugar that is the white crystal most culpable in hypertension and cardiovascular disease."[8]

Low sodium intake has been correlated with increased mortality in some populations[9], especially among those not suffering from obesity or insulin resistance. And among ketogenic or carnivore eaters, salt becomes even more vital.

Dr. Frassetto's work highlights that a low sodium-to-potassium ratio, not sodium alone, is more predictive of hypertension[10]. And salt sensitivity, too, varies with genetics; individuals of African descent, for example, tend to exhibit heightened responsiveness to sodium fluctuations. When processed food replaces real salt and mineral-dense meat, the ratio collapses, and pathology follows.

Salt was framed for a murder sugar committed. It was the scapegoat of the processed food priesthood. It was the mineral of meat, and that alone made it suspect.

But salt's truth lives not just in labs… it pulses in the stories we've forgotten.

The Butcher's Salt Box

The salt box was wood. Oak, darkened with grease. It sat beside the butcher's sink, its lid worn smooth from three generations of fingers.

His grandfather had called it "the memory chest." A pinch of Maldon on raw liver. A ritual. A sacrament.

He used to watch as a child - how the old man sliced, salted, and chewed. "You eat it first," he'd say. "Before you cook. So, you remember where it came from. Salt it first, so you know it still lives."

Years passed. The butcher's grandson became a man. He forgot the salt. Forgot the taste of blood. Ate plants and powders. Guzzled green smoothies. Got sick.

When the diagnosis came, it wasn't a surprise. What surprised him was what he remembered in the quiet. The weight of the salt box. The sting of a flake on his tongue. The taste of blood beneath the mineral.

The warmth that followed - not of spice, but of truth. He returned to flesh. He salted it. And the memory returned with it. He did not heal with herbs. He healed with a crystal. And with memory.

The Vampire's Crystal

The vampire does not fear salt. He requires it. To preserve blood. To protect fire. To anchor flesh to instinct.

Salt is not merely a crystal. It is a covenant. It holds the contract between predator and prey, between kill and memory. It dries meat for the journey. It cauterizes wounds. It wards off decay. It stops the rot.

Salt is the shadow of the sea left behind in the blood. Modern man fears salt like he fears blood, because both remind him of what he's lost. Salt is not the enemy of life. Salt is the proof that it still flows.

Cord and Crystal

She gave birth alone, kneeling in ash. The wolves circled, but they did not come close. The fire held them back.

When the child crowned, she bit the leather and screamed.

After the cord was cut with stone, she reached into the pouch of crushed rock. Salt from the well. A gift from the old ones. She rubbed it into the cord. Onto her skin. Into the ashes where the blood had fallen. "So, he will not rot," she whispered. "So, she would not forget." Salt sealed the covenant between life and death, a promise against decay, etched in ash and blood.

The Ritual Reclaimed

To salt like an ancestor is to remember like one. You don't need precision scales or electrolyte apps. The body speaks. On a carnivore diet, salting to taste is a sign of restored instinct. There is no one-size-fits-all sodium rule, but there is a forgotten wisdom that returns when the tongue is honest.

How to salt like a predator: Use real salt: grey, pink, or white, but from earth or sea, not factories. (Celtic, Maldon, Himalayan.) Himalayan salt contains 84 trace minerals that nourish adrenal resilience.

Salt your fat, not just your muscle. Fat carries the mineral well. Add salt to your broth, to your raw liver, to your rituals. Use your hands. Feel the flakes. Honor the kill. Ritualize the act. Make it deliberate. Sacred. Sensory.

Salt is not a flavor enhancer. Salt is an awakening agent. To salt the flesh is to mark it as sacred. To salt your food is to remember the fire. To salt your life is to preserve the predator within.

Salt the kill. Keep the code. In the end, it was never about sodium. It was about remembering.

Chapter 8

The Undying Mind - Why Vampires Don't Get Alzheimer's

You forget what you want to remember, and you remember what you want to forget.

A vampire never forgets.

Centuries pass. Empires crumble. Faces wither. Still, he remembers. The name of a lover whispered in the flicker of torchlight. The scent of blood spilled on Roman stone. The cold thrill of a thousand moonlit hunts. A mind sharpened by centuries, unspoiled by fog.

Modern man, by contrast, forgets where he parked the car. We accept it, age brings decline. Memory fades. Confusion comes. The cruel laugh of Alzheimer's haunts our family trees. "It's genetic," they say. "It's just aging." But what if it isn't?

What if it's a dietary curse? A metabolic betrayal? What if the vampire's enduring mind isn't fantasy, but a clue?

Strip away the cloak and fangs, and what do you see? A creature that fasts. A creature that feeds rarely, with precision. A creature that never touches sugar. He lives in ketosis. He does not graze. And his brain does not rot.

The Glucose Trap

The brain is a greedy organ. It devours 20% of your energy while weighing just 2% of your body. In the modern world, that energy is glucose… sugar. We eat it constantly. We sip it, snack it, and inject it into every processed bite. Our brains are tethered to it like a lifeline turned leash. But in Alzheimer's disease, the brain starts rejecting its only fix.

Long before diagnosis, neurons in the hippocampus - the seat of memory - stop metabolizing glucose properly. They become insulin-resistant. The fuel is there, but the gate is closed. This is why some researchers call Alzheimer's "type 3 diabetes"[1]. The lights flicker. Memory fades. The self dissolves.

Glucose Hypometabolism: The Brain Starves First

Even before the first forgotten name or misplaced key, the brain's energy crisis begins. PET scans reveal that glucose metabolism declines in the hippocampus and other memory-critical regions years before symptoms emerge[2]. This isn't just a side effect of aging. It's an early red flag.

One study found a 17-24% reduction in cerebral glucose uptake in Alzheimer's patients compared to healthy peers[3]. Starvation of the brain doesn't wait for dementia. It lays the path for it.

Why Memory Is Metabolic

Memory is not magic. It's infrastructure. To encode, store, and recall, the brain demands high-octane energy. Each memory requires ATP to fire synapses, generate dendritic spines, maintain structural integrity.

Glucose, in the inflamed modern brain, fails to deliver. Ketones do not. Ketones bypass insulin resistance, fuel neurons directly, and generate more ATP per unit than glucose[4]. They burn cleaner. They silence chaos. They feed not just survival, but signal, strength, and story.

Memory is metabolic. The mind is made of meals.

Lucien Has Not Eaten in Three Days

Lucien waits in the shadows of an old chapel. Three days since he last fed. His senses are sharpened, not dulled. He can hear the slow heartbeat of a man two floors above. His vision pulses with detail. But it's his memory that cuts the sharpest edge.

He remembers the weight of coins in Florence. The rhythm of a German soldier's boots in 1916. The precise shape of a broken oath. Lucien is in ketosis.

His brain is not declining. It is ascending, fed by the clean fire of fat and fasting. No fog. No confusion. No forgetting.

While no diet guarantees immunity, ketosis significantly lowers Alzheimer's risk factors, especially when initiated early, before significant neuronal loss.

Ketones: Fuel of the Undying

When humans fast, or eat like predators, the liver produces ketones: beta-hydroxybutyrate (βHB), acetoacetate, and acetone. These are not backup fuel. They are ancestral flame. And they don't just keep neurons alive. They make them better:

- They boost mitochondria, increasing ATP while reducing oxidative stress[5].
- They silence inflammation, blocking the NLRP3 inflammasome[6].
- They flip genetic switches, activating FOXO3A and PGC-1α for longevity[7].
- They clean the wreckage. Though amyloid plaques remain a biomarker, emerging research emphasizes neuroinflammation and tau tangles as equal drivers of decline[8]. Ketones restore transport proteins like LRP1 and P-glycoprotein to help clear debris[9].

Modern medicine tries antibodies. The vampire uses time and fat. While ketones efficiently fuel 60–70% of the brain during fasting states, certain brain regions retain some glucose dependence.

This reminds us that metabolic flexibility, not dogma, is nature's way.

BDNF: The Flame That Rebuilds

Ketones raise brain-derived neurotrophic factor (BDNF)[10], nature's neural Miracle-Gro. It supports neurogenesis, strengthens synapses, and enhances learning. In one mouse study, βHB increased hippocampal BDNF expression by over 50%[11].

A brain that runs on ketones doesn't just resist decay. It evolves. Vampires don't just remember. They resist erosion through ancestral fire.

The Carnivore Remembers

In Dracula, the Count recalls Jonathan Harker's scent years after his visit. Every detail - his voice, gait, the shape of his thoughts - locked in memory. This is not merely romantic horror. This is cognitive clarity fueled by constraint.

And Dracula is not alone. Nosferatu, the silent one, fasts between feedings for weeks, saying nothing, moving little. His mind does not drift. His purpose remains fixed. The lich remembers ancient spells. The revenant returns with perfect vengeance.

Like the vampire, these beings defy decay through metabolic mastery. They do not snack. They do not sip sugar. They do not forget.

Dracula's Dream

Three centuries ago. A girl with jasmine in her hair. A first kill. The scent of sweat and petals. The pulse at her throat. He remembers not in outline, but in texture. Her breath. Her eyes. Her fear. Not even time could blur the memory. For Dracula, the past is not past. It is lit, alive, encoded in blood.

The Blood-Brain Barrier

In Alzheimer's, the blood-brain barrier (BBB), the fortress between blood and thought, starts to break. Glycation and inflammation tear it open. The wrong molecules get in. The right ones can't get out. Ketones patch the wall.

βHB restores the integrity of the BBB by upregulating tight-junction proteins like claudin-5 and occludin[12]. These gatekeeper proteins form the brain's security system, locking out toxins and preserving memory.

Signs You're Fueling Like a Vampire

- You skip breakfast and feel sharper, not sluggish[16].
- You crave meat and salt, not muffins.
- You wake before your alarm, clear and calm.
- You remember names, details, and old dreams.
- You don't fear hunger, you hunt it.
- You feel ancient and focused.
- You enjoy silence. Darkness. Solitude.

How to Think Like a Vampire

- Begin with 14 - 16 hour fasts. Graduate to 20+.
- Eat once a day, and feast well.
- Choose fatty meat. Prioritize brain-fueling nutrients: choline (liver, eggs), DHA (fish roe), B12 (ruminant meat).
- Balance electrolytes, use salt, magnesium, and potassium when starting.
- Move in sunlight. Sleep in darkness.
- Avoid seed oils. Sip salt.
- Aim for βHB levels of 1.0 - 3.0 mmol/L.
- Do not graze. Do not sugar. Do not forget.
- Remember: ketosis is foundational, but so are sleep, light rhythms, and toxin avoidance.

Modern Evidence: Trials and Transformation

In a 2020 clinical trial, patients with mild cognitive impairment who consumed a ketogenic drink daily showed measurable improvements in executive function and memory[13].

And in one extraordinary case, Dr. Mary Newport fed her husband MCT oil when his Alzheimer's progressed. His cognition began to return within days[14]. Ketones weren't abstract. They were his lifeline.

A 2018 study confirmed this effect in broader trials[17]. And in 2021, another study found that ketogenic diets improved verbal memory and daily function in Alzheimer's patients after just 12 weeks[15]. The fog lifted. The fire returned.

The Forgotten Man

Arthur sits in his chair, staring at the screen. He reaches for his tea, forgetting it's already in his hand. He once lectured in philosophy. Now he forgets his daughter's name. His breakfast is toast. His fuel is sugar. His neurons starve. His mind dims. He is not undead. He is unremembered.

Lucien vs. Arthur: A Comparison

Lucien fasts. Arthur snacks. Lucien fuels with blood and fat. Arthur eats toast and tea. Lucien's brain sharpens with silence. Arthur's fogs with sugar. Lucien remembers. Arthur forgets.

The Resurrection of the Mind

You don't need to drink blood to think like a vampire. You just need to stop poisoning your brain with glucose. Return to meat. Return to fat. Return to fasting. Let your brain burn clean. Let your memory rise from the grave.

Salt stabilizes the spark. Fat feeds the flame. Ketones remember. The blood remembers. And so will you. Feed like a predator. Fast like a mystic. Remember like the undead.

Chapter 9

The Suntan Vampire

How Flesh, Fat, and Firelight Forged Our Sun-Hardened Skin

He was first spotted in Ibiza. Not hiding from the sun but absorbing it. Shirt off, shoulders bronze, sipping bone broth from a battered steel thermos. Locals whispered he never ate paella. Never aged. Never wore sunscreen. They called him… The Suntan Vampire.

He wasn't like the others. No basement lair. No velvet-lined coffin. He lived by the shore, hunted at dawn, grilled liver under moonlight. And while the crowds staggered beneath UV umbrellas, smearing white pastes onto their wilting skin, he stood bare-chested, golden, and untouchable.

Some say there were two kinds of vampires. The nightwalkers: pale, haunted, cursed. And the fire-fed: those rare ancestors who stood bare to the blaze, skin fortified by blood and brine. Their lineage whispered through myth and marrow. The Suntan Vampire was one of them.

The Myth of the Pale Predator

For centuries, we imagined vampires as pale and photophobic. But what if we misunderstood the myth? What if the original predator wasn't repelled by the sun but thrived in it? What if sunlight wasn't the enemy… civilization was?

Vampires were once apex creatures of flesh, firelight, and instinct. They feasted on blood, not because they were monsters but because they remembered the ancestral fuel. Today, our modern undead are not the sun-averse creatures of gothic fiction. They are the pasty, inflamed descendants of grain-fed serfs. Vampirism wasn't a curse. It was a remnant. You do not photosynthesize. You metabolize.

The truth is simple: when you eat like a predator, the sun does not burn you. It anoints you.

Your Skin Is Not Decoration, It's Armor

Skin is your shield. It is not passive. It is not cosmetic. It is alive.

Modern medicine reduces it to a dermatological surface, but skin is a dynamic immune organ. It senses. It synthesizes. It secretes. It regenerates. And when properly nourished, it defends.

Its outermost layer, the stratum corneum, or outer brickwork of the skin, is composed of keratinized cells embedded in a lipid matrix, much like bricks set in mortar. That mortar is made of ceramides (your skin's natural moisturizers), cholesterol, and free fatty acids, all of which require a high-fat, nutrient-dense diet to maintain[4].

When these layers are intact, UV rays are met with resilience. When they're built on industrial seed oils like soybean or corn, sugar, and stress hormones, the sun becomes your enemy. In contrast, traditional fats, animal-based and even some monounsaturated oils like olive oil - are more stable in the skin.

The UV Spectrum: Predator vs Prey

Sunlight carries two main ultraviolet weapons: UVA and UVB.

- **UVA** penetrates deeper into the dermis, causing oxidative stress and collagen breakdown (wrinkles, sagging, ageing).
- **UVB** is responsible for surface burning, but also for the synthesis of Vitamin D_3 via cholesterol in the skin[4].

Your reaction to these depends on your internal terrain. If your lipid profile is balanced, your mitochondrial defenses strong, and your skin nourished, UV radiation can be tolerated and even beneficial. If your membranes are built from linoleic acid, processed sugar, and stress, you will blister like a paper vampire[7].

And while metabolic health reduces burn risk, prolonged exposure, especially for lighter Fitzpatrick skin types, still calls for wisdom. Shade, hats and timing. Even the old vampires knew. When the sun rose high, they sought caves or cloaks. Wisdom is not weakness.

Eat to Endure the Light: Nutrient Defense Systems

1. **Retinol (Real Vitamin A):** Not beta-carotene, but the active form found in liver and animal fat. Retinol upregulates skin cell turnover, boosts antioxidant enzyme activity, and assists in nucleotide excision repair, the mechanism by which damaged DNA is patched after UV exposure[1].

2. **Zinc:** Abundant in red meat and oysters, zinc plays a pivotal role in metalloenzyme regulation, immune signaling, and the control of inflammatory cytokines. It also directly assists in the reconstruction of UV-damaged cells[2].

3. **Saturated Fat and Cholesterol**: Essential for ceramide synthesis, barrier function, and skin flexibility[4]. Cholesterol is also the raw material from which your body produces vitamin D_3 in the skin, this is via a compound called 7-dehydrocholesterol. A cholesterol precursor that catches UVB like a solar antenna.

And cholesterol is more than that. It is the original conduit between blood and light. In the predator's body, sunlight is not something to fear. It's something to metabolize. Cholesterol turns solar radiation into calcitriol, the hormonal sunbeam that regulates immunity, inflammation, and mood.

The vampire glows not because of SPF, but because of fuel.

4. **Glycine and Collagen**: Derived from bone broth, tendons, and skin, these amino acids support dermal density and help resist UV-induced collagen degradation.

5. **Omega-3 Fatty Acids**: Found in fatty cuts of meat, egg yolks, and wild fish, omega-3s help stabilize cell membranes, reduce inflammation, and modulate the skin's response to UV stress. Studies show that regular intake may reduce UV-induced damage and support a more robust tanning response[6]. While plant-based sources like flax and chia contain ALA, their conversion to the protective EPA/DHA forms is minimal.

6. **Magnesium and Selenium**: Magnesium, abundant in red meat, activates vitamin D in the liver and kidneys. Selenium, found in kidney and seafood, fuels glutathione - the skin's internal sun shield.

A plant-based diet struggles to support these systems. Anti-nutrients like phytic acid, oxalates, and lectins interfere with mineral absorption. Grains deplete zinc. Seed oils oxidize in the skin[7]. Carbohydrates promote glycation, damaging the very collagen that keeps you youthful.

Photoprotection Is Metabolic, Not Cosmetic

The cosmetics industry wants you to believe protection comes from tubes. But a layer of SPF is not a substitute for cellular fortitude.

Photoprotection begins with the mitochondria, your cellular energy generators. UV exposure generates reactive oxygen species (ROS), which are normally neutralized by enzymes like superoxide dismutase and glutathione peroxidase. These antioxidant systems are upregulated in fat-adapted, low-insulin individuals, such as those eating carnivore or ketogenic diets[3].

In one human study, supplementing with nicotinamide (vitamin B3) reduced the rate of non-melanoma skin cancer recurrence by over 20%[5]. While nicotinamide is also found in mushrooms and legumes, meat delivers it in its most bioavailable and complete form, where it's already packaged with cofactors your skin understands.

This is not a dismissal of all sunscreens. High-altitude glare, long exposures, or prior damage may warrant temporary use. But for the metabolically rewilded, protection begins within.

The Sunlit Alchemy of Cholesterol

When UVB strikes your skin, it interacts with 7-dehydrocholesterol, a compound synthesized from dietary cholesterol. This is not a bonus feature. It is a central function of your skin. The result? Pre-vitamin D_3, which converts into active calcitriol, a steroid hormone that helps regulate over 1,000 genes, including those involved in immunity, inflammation, and cell repair.

But this solar alchemy requires animal fat, not just for the cholesterol, but for the transport of fat-soluble cofactors:

- Vitamin K2, found in egg yolks and liver, helps shuttle calcium to the bones.
- Magnesium, found in meat, activates vitamin D.
- Selenium, from organ meats and seafood, strengthens intracellular defenses.
- Tallow and suet, rich in stearic acid, support mitochondrial energy output, enhancing your skin's resilience.

A carnivore's body doesn't just tolerate sunlight. It's designed to complete the reaction. Be the kind of carnivore who doesn't fear the sun... feed on it.

Ancestral Skin Was Sun-Hardened

The fossil record doesn't reveal many moisturizer routines. But it does show something else: bone thickness, collagen strength, and high-density nutrient markers in early hominids who lived beneath the sun and ate animals nose-to-tail. We didn't fear the sun. We evolved with it.

Dark-skinned ancestors in equatorial Africa developed high melanin levels to regulate intense UVB exposure. Northern carnivores developed efficient cholesterol-driven vitamin D systems and robust fat layers for insulation and resilience[4].

And in both cases, their ability to tan and adapt to the sun was not random. It was built on stable insulin levels, high fat intake, and low inflammation. When you eat like a predator, melanin works with you, not against you.

Post-agricultural populations show striking biological decline: shorter stature, porous bone, increased anemia, and collagen loss - visible proof that grains traded resilience for fragility[8].

And yet, some cultures found balance. Mediterranean populations, for instance, buffered their grain consumption with seafood, olive oil, and organ meats, avoiding the total collapse seen in other grain-heavy civilizations. Still, many traded liver for lentils, marrow for millet. They surrendered radiant, fortified skin for dermatological fragility.

And our oldest myths remembered. Consider: Ra, the solar god of Egypt. Helios, the flaming charioteer. Sol Invictu, the unconquered sun. These were not idle metaphors. They were metabolic truths wrapped in ritual. They worshipped the light because the light sustained them.

The Suntan Vampire Returns

He returned not to Ibiza, but to a rooftop in Berlin. It was mid-July. Tourists crammed into cafés, fanning themselves with oat milk receipts.

He stood still, bare-chested. Skin bronze, veins like braided cords. A young woman offered him a straw hat and a bottle of mineral sunscreen.

He looked at her, amused. "I don't burn," he said again. "I feed on the light." He pulled a marrow bone from his satchel, cracked it on the rail, and drank. The sunrise split across the skyline… and he laughed.

Some say he disappeared. Others say he never left. He just changed his name to… Duncan.

The Modern Vampire

Let's be truthful. Those who avoid meat often report the very symptoms the vampire once carried: pale skin, fatigue, sun sensitivity, and a need to retreat from the light. They do not feast on blood. They leak vitality. Their glow dimmed not by nature, but by nutrition. They are not damned. They're deficient. And they can recover.

Live Like the Predator You Were Born To Be

The vampire, in this new light, is not a monster. He is an ancestral echo. A symbol of what we once were, and what we might become again. Like our bronze stranger on the rooftop, marrow in hand, laughing at the dawn, you too can reclaim the glow that once marked the hunter.

Be bronze. Be bold. Be carnivore. Be the kind of vampire who doesn't fear the sun. Feed on it.

Chapter 10

The Fat Phobia Ritual

We didn't just lose our appetite for fat. We buried it in guilt.

Heart Attack on a Plate

Imagine this: you're at a brunch table with friends, and your plate glistens with unapologetic glory, streaky bacon, eggs fried in butter, perhaps even a smug little dollop of bone marrow.

You take your first bite. Enter the Concerned One. "That," they declare, "looks like a heart attack on a plate." They don't even blink. You, however, are caught mid-chew with a strip of bacon like a guilty weapon in your mouth.

Congratulations. You've just stumbled into one of the last socially acceptable public shaming... fat consumption! Fat, you see, isn't just a macronutrient. In modern Western society, it's a moral failing. A dietary sin. Eating it in public is a subversive act, like lighting a cigar in a vegan yoga studio. And this isn't just about the food. It's about what fat represents. Pleasure. Decadence. Rebellion. Something primal and wild that civilization has been trying to neuter for decades.

Ancel's Curse and the Cult of Fat Fear

To understand the roots of this ritualistic fear, we must return to a man whose mustache still silently judges you from nutritional hell: Ancel Keys.

In the 1950s, Keys gave birth to what might be the most consequential dietary blunder in modern history. The lipid hypothesis claimed saturated fat caused heart disease. His infamous Seven Countries Study cherry-picked data, ignoring cultures like the Maasai and Inuit whose fat-heavy diets didn't result in arterial carnage. He also excluded nations like France and Switzerland, where high-fat diets coincided with low rates of cardiovascular disease.

While Keys dismissed them, these cultures didn't just eat fat. They revered it. The Inuit shared seal blubber like sacramental wine, believing akutuq (whipped fat and berries) carried ancestral wisdom. The Maasai blended blood and milk into kule naoto, a warrior's fuel of courage. In Norse sagas, gods gained strength from Odin's sacred butter. Fat wasn't feared; it was worshiped as life condensed.

Modern fat phobia didn't just pathologize lipids. It severed a sacred thread to our metabolic ancestry. But Keys had charm, influence, and the political will behind him. Governments listened. Fat was demonized. Carbs were canonized.

By the 1980s, the USDA food pyramid rose like a nutritional ziggurat. Grains formed its holy base. "Heart-healthy" margarine sat upon its golden capstone. Fat, especially saturated fat, was exiled like a heretic.

Schoolchildren were fed on pyramid logic: low-fat milk cartons, dry turkey sandwiches, and food posters listing fat alongside cigarettes. Doctors repeated the script. Supermarkets rebranded their shelves. Snack bars, cereals, frozen dinners, all proudly labelled "low fat," as if that alone was a virtue. The pyramid wasn't just policy. It was culture.

I once watched my niece's health class dissect a "bad food" poster. A cartoon heart wept over bacon. A villainous stick of butter twirled its mustache. When a boy asked why his Inuit cousin ate seal fat, the teacher snapped: "That's their tradition. We know better."

Here's the tragedy: we don't teach nutrition; we teach dogma. Children learn fat equals failure. Fat equals shame. And by the time they're adults, they'll police brunch tables with the same fervor as pyramid priests.

We didn't just fear fat. We ritualized its absence. We equated its presence with death, and its rejection with moral superiority.

Fatness, especially in women of color, was pathologized long before cholesterol entered the chat. The pyramid didn't merely moralize fat. It mapped metabolism onto a colonial blueprint.

The Ladder and the Monkeys

There's a classic behavioral experiment. A group of monkeys are placed in a cage with a ladder and bananas on top. When one monkey climbs, the whole group is sprayed with cold water. Soon, no one climbs.

One by one, the monkeys are replaced. New monkeys try the ladder, and the group beats them back, even though the punishment no longer comes. Eventually, none of the monkeys in the cage have ever been sprayed. But none of them will climb. Ask them why, and the answer would be: "That's just the way it's done."

That, dear reader, is Western dietary culture. We no longer question fat phobia. We inherit it. We don't need studies, just social cues. Fat is no longer a nutrient. It's a taboo.

Confessions of a Clean Eater

- Day 1: I bought low-fat hummus. It tasted like beige and regret.
- Day 3: I skipped the yolks again. Just the whites. It's like eating sadness in sponge form.
- Day 5: I used canola oil spray on my kale chips. I miss chewing.
- Day 12: I dreamt I licked a spoonful of beef tallow. I woke up ashamed… and salivating.
- Day 16: I relapsed. Bone marrow and butter. It was glorious. I am unclean. I am free.

Eat Clean. Die Empty

Your arteries will thank you. Your hormones will vanish. And your soul will be morally spotless. "Tired of that heavy, primal instinct to feast? Suppress it with our new zero-fat Food-Like Substance™. Now with 0% guilt, 0% cholesterol, and 100% shelf life."

Low-fat. High virtue. All sacrifice. For indulgence is sin. Hunger is holiness.

Vampires Don't Eat Granola

Let's shift. Consider the archetypal vampire: pale, elegant, eternally alive. A creature of the night who thrives on blood, fat, and flesh. No oat milk. No quinoa. No salad dressing made with industrial seed oils. When vampires feed, it's carnivorous, caloric, and deeply intermittent.

They don't snack. They don't graze. They feast.

The Vampire Who Feared the Feast

There once was a vampire named Lucien. For centuries, he fed on warriors, hunters, the wild. Their blood was thick with life. It made him strong.

But time passed. The modern world came. People got softer, sweeter... their blood more like syrup than strength.

Lucien complied. He followed the health advice, feeding only on joggers who drank skimmed milk and ate dry toast. Their blood was light. It was pure. It was wrong. He began to lose his memory. His senses dulled. His reflection no longer scared him. Even the night forgot his name.

One evening, in a dim city park, Lucien collapsed. He hadn't fed, not truly, in months. A carnivore couple found him. Revived him with tallow, marrow, and ribeye. He awoke confused, then enlightened. "You weren't feeding," they said. "You were starving yourself on fear."

From that night forward, Lucien fed differently. He hunted unapologetically. He feasted. He got stronger. Sharper. His blood turned dark again, rich with mitochondrial fire. BDNF sparked in his brain like lightning across a long-forgotten map.

Eventually, he began writing a book. He called it *Blood and Bone*. And this time, he made sure it was marbled with truth.

When the Body Says No

You can live without fat. But only for a while. Then the body begins to whisper. Then it begins to scream.

- You lose your period.
- Your skin cracks.
- Your thoughts slow.
- Your libido vanishes.

- Your sleep falters.
- You're cold. Always cold.
- You look 'fit'... but feel like you're fading.

Fat fuels hormones. It insulates neurons. It protects against inflammation. Without it, the body withers in slow, socially approved starvation.

Leptin, the hormone that tells your brain you're nourished, plummets. Ghrelin, the hunger hormone, misfires, driving you to snack endlessly. Cholesterol, the raw material for sex hormones, becomes a scapegoat instead of the hero it truly is, like blaming bricks for a crumbling cathedral[1] [2].

To lose fat is not to gain virtue. To reject fat is not to become clean. You do not become holy by starving your mitochondria.

Fat Facts They Don't Teach in School

Let's gut the myths. Here's what peer-reviewed science actually shows:

- Fat burns clean. Ketones (like β-hydroxybutyrate) generate less oxidative stress than glucose. This reduces inflammation and preserves mitochondria[3].
- Ketones protect the brain. They improve cognitive function, reduce brain fog, and may defend against Alzheimer's by increasing mitochondrial efficiency[4].
- Fat doesn't clog your arteries. Sugar and inflammation do. Small, dense LDL particles, the real villains in

atherosclerosis, are elevated by insulin, not dietary fat[5].

- Industrial seed oils like soybean and canola are the real dietary bomb. Their oxidized linoleic acid contributes to systemic inflammation and mitochondrial dysfunction[6].

- You don't get fat from fat. You get fat from insulin. Fat doesn't spike insulin. Carbs do[7].

- Recent studies continue to vindicate low-carbohydrate diets, showing improvements in cardiovascular risk and metabolic resilience[8].

- Even saturated fat, long demonized, has been reassessed as not independently linked to cardiovascular mortality[9].

- And context matters. Whole-food animal fats behave differently than processed, sugar-laced meats. The food matrix matters.

Mental Reprogramming Required

Even now, with science stacked like slabs of brisket in fat's favor, many of us still flinch.

- Cooking with butter? "Just a little."
- Scooping marrow onto steak? "Isn't that excessive?"
- Finishing a plate of ribeye and yolks? "Have I overdone it?" No. You haven't. But your conditioning has.

Take Elena. After 15 years of low-fat orthorexia, she wept over her first ribeye. "I feel like I'm betraying everything I was taught," she whispered.

Six months later? Her arthritis pain vanished. Her hormones rebooted. At her wedding, she served bone marrow toast and laughed as her mother gasped. "This," she told me, "Is my rebellion."

The Gospel of Grains and the Discomfort of Doubt

Many of us didn't just follow the low-fat gospel. We evangelize it. We warned others off butter. We felt virtuous with skimmed milk. We rolled our eyes at steak lovers like they were medieval gluttons.

To accept fat is healthy isn't just to revise your diet. It's to renounce your nutritional religion. The very metric we use to define "health," BMI, was designed by Adolphe Quetelet to measure average white male bodies. It was never a tool of health. Yet we wield it like gospel.

Cognitive dissonance is not just discomfort. It's identity collapse. Changing what you eat is one thing. Changing who you think you are? That's war.

But here's the truth: There is no shame in waking up. There is only power in pivoting. It takes courage to say, "I was wrong, and now I know better." That isn't failure. That is evolution. And evolution, as any vampire will tell you, favors those who adapt.

Burn the Ladder. Reclaim the Feast.

Picture the monkeys. The ladder. The fear. Now picture yourself, with a fork. The fat is there. The feast is ready. The ladder still looms, built of old ads, outdated studies, and the voices of your mother, your doctor, and your inner food cop. You hesitate. And then… you climb. You eat. You burn the damn ladder.

Go to your fridge. Throw away the light yogurt. Open the butter. Taste it. Eat it with your fingers. Say this out loud:

"FAT IS NOT MY ENEMY. FAT IS MY FIRE."

Chapter 11

The Predator's Pantry: Why We Hunted And Not Gathered

Vampires don't pick berries… they hunt.

The Lie of the Berry Picker

You were told we were gatherers. That for millennia, we quietly plucked fruit from trees, knelt to pull roots, and foraged like herbivorous monks awaiting the accidental invention of bacon.

But that is not how predators live. And you were not born from passive hands and plant-stained mouths. You were carved by hunger. Forged in pursuit.

We were not gatherers who occasionally hunted. We were hunters who occasionally gathered. To gather is to wait. To hunt is to decide. And the vampire does not pick berries.

Our Predator's Anatomy

Your body remembers:

- Eyes facing forward, not for scanning leaves, but for tracking motion.
- Achilles tendons built for running prey to collapse.

- Sweat glands erupting across skin like a living cooling system.
- A stomach acid pH like a vulture's.
- A short intestinal tract, designed for meat, not fiber.
- The ability to store vast energy, then expend it in a burst of pursuit.

You don't evolve these traits for nibbling blueberries. The human body is an apex predator's machine: designed not just to run, but to endure. We are the only primates that pant. We can outrun antelope, not in speed, but in time. While the prey gasps, we breathe. While they rest, we stalk.

We were made not just to hunt, but to win. "Humans are the only primates adapted for endurance running, capable of pursuing animals for hours under the sun."[1] And what did that running feed? A brain. One that grew to devour the world.

The Brain on Meat

Meat made the mind. It's not just a poetic flourish… it's a metabolic fact.

The expensive tissue hypothesis[2] tells us that the brain's energy cost had to be offset by something. That "something" was meat: calorie-dense, bioavailable, nutrient-rich flesh that required less chewing, less processing, and less gut real estate.

Fire finished the job. Fire made nutrients more bioavailable, reduced chewing time, and freed our ancestors' jaws, and mind, for language. Fire turned sinew to sustenance. It turned bones to broth, and time to thought. "The fallback food of starving humans has never been meat. It's plants."[3]

The anthropological record speaks clearly. Even a modest deer yields around 50,000 calories, enough to feed 20 people for 3 days. A mammoth? Over 3.6 million[4]. One clean kill could feed a tribe and allow for rest, ritual, and regeneration. Plants required constant foraging, detoxification, and yielded far less per hour of effort. "Among the !Kung, hunting was not just sustenance. It was status, story, and spiritual calling."[5] When meat was secured, the tribe transformed.

The Parable of the Empty Hunt

In San tradition, a failed hunt is not just disappointing. It's sacred. The emptiness teaches patience. The slow drumbeat of learning. The worth of the feast to come.

Lucien remembered this patience. He'd tracked rebels through frozen Baltic forests for weeks, moving only at dusk. The kill was never rushed. It was earned. And when the hunter returns with meat? The ritual begins. "Even a mammoth could sustain generations."[4]

Not with scarcity. With sacrifice. Not with greed. With gratitude.

The Fire That Feeds

When the meat returns, the fire center ignites more than wood. It lights memory. Ceremony. Myth.

It is here that the feminine power reappears, not in prey capture, but in everything that followed: the cutting, the distributing, the feeding, the flame. Women knew who needed liver, who had bled last moon, who bore the child of the warrior who would not return. They fed the future. In matriarchal societies like the Mosuo, women held the knives, and the power flowed with the fat.

While men often pursued large game, women tracked smaller prey, set traps, and in societies from the Agta to the Amazon, wielded spears themselves. Agta women in the Philippines have been documented contributing up to 30% of large game meat. Even female chimpanzees hunt red colobus monkeys - suggesting predation runs deep in our shared lineage.

The fire was not gendered. It was the tribe's command center. And with the kill came story. Meat built bodies. Blood built story.

Predator's Toolkit

To hunt is to track. To track is to think. Our hands don't just throw spears... they spin stories. The same neural wiring that calculates a gazelle's path plots a parable's climax.

Our brains reward the chase. fMRI scans show modern hunters experiencing dopamine surges not when eating meat, but when tracking prey. This neural wiring explains why gamers lose hours in virtual forests, and why Lucien's Baltic pursuit felt like prayer. The predator's high isn't bloodlust. It's focus forged by evolution[10].

When anthropologists surveyed 229 hunter-gatherer societies, they found something radical: not one was primarily vegetarian. Even in plant-rich environments, meat comprised 45 - 80% of calories. The Aché of Paraguay got 78% from game. The Hiwi of Venezuela tracked peccary while ignoring ripe fruit. For the Nunamiut Eskimo, famine food meant plants, not caribou[12]. "A deer may yield around 50,000 calories of nutrient-dense meat and fat… They do not sprint - they walk, watch, and wear down the prey under a pitiless sun."

Yes, we processed plants when prey was scarce, but at great energetic cost, and never as a preferred replacement for animal fat and protein. Plants were fallback fuel, not foundational fire. Even bones were cracked open for the red gold of marrow… nature's fat-soaked signature.

"Persistence hunting isn't a fable. It's fossilized in heel strikes and sweat glands."[6] In modern times, !Xo San trackers still run kudu to collapse under 40°C heat, covering miles barefoot.[6]

Beyond the Mammal

The carnivore strategy didn't end at land beasts. We hunted fish. We speared eels. We cracked shellfish on stone. "The vampire does not care if the blood is warm or cold... only that it flows."

At Blombos Cave, 100,000 years ago, our ancestors left behind heaps of shellfish middens: fossilized evidence of seafood that fed our growing brains. From the sea came DHA - brain fuel unlike any plant could offer. "Even in matriarchal forager bands, protein distribution determined status. Control of the meat meant command of the moment."[7]

Return of the Predator

Here's the irony: contemporary foragers with access to Western foods still choose meat. When the Aché got metal tools, they hunted more, not less. When the Hadza tried farming, they abandoned it within years. "Maize makes us weak," one elder told me.

Our DNA hasn't forgotten what our culture denies: plants sustain, but meat makes us alive.

To hunt like a predator isn't savagery. It's honoring the life taken. It's rejecting factory farms. It's wasting nothing. It's remembering what you are. We were prey, yes, but we evolved to hunt back harder. "The predator must not only kill... it must remember."[8]

The Feast That Forged Us

You don't paint a carrot on a cave wall. You paint the hunt. The moment the blood met stone. The marrow met flame. The tribe rose in voice and firelight. Because the feast that forged us human was not a salad. It was meat.

Hunter-Gatherer Macronutrient Ratios

- **Nunamiut (Alaska):** 99% of calories from meat, primarily caribou. Plants only consumed during famine.
- **!Kung (Kalahari):** 65% meat intake, focusing on antelope. Supplemented with mongongo nuts.
- **Aché (Paraguay):** 78% of calories from game like peccary. Plants (e.g., palm starch) used strategically.

Chapter 12

Why Nature Never Served Protein Alone

The flame was in the fat. The strength was in the flesh. The kill was never meant to be split.

The Forgotten Law

They say you should eat lean. Trim the meat. Discard the skin. Separate the yolk. Worship the number on the label that says protein, and fear the one that whispers fat.

But nature never served protein alone. Not to wolves. Not to bears. Not to the child that suckled at the breast and tasted both cream and casein, both fuel and form.

The body was not designed for lean. It was designed for the kill, complete. The predator does not carve the kill by macronutrient. It bites. It swallows. It remembers.

And yet we live in a culture that split the flesh from the flame. That drained the marrow, skimmed the cream, praised the egg white and poured the yolk down the drain. A society that calls fat indulgent, and lean meat noble, as if cutting the kill in half could preserve the body whole.

But when you tear protein from fat, something else is torn too: Memory. Fertility. Fire.

The Man Who Ate Only Muscle

He was strong, but dying. You could see every sinew beneath his skin. Dry cords of flesh. Tightly packed precision. And yet his eyes blurred when he stood. His thoughts scattered like snow on a thawed hill. He could no longer hold his daughter without trembling.

He had eaten only muscle. Egg whites. Chicken breast. Tuna cans in spring water. Protein powder that clung to the sides of plastic shaker bottles like chalk in a gymnasium grave. He feared fat like a curse. Thought it would soften him, slow him, make him weak.

But fat is not the enemy. Fat is what fuels the hunt.

When he collapsed, they called it overtraining. When he lost his sex drive, they blamed cortisol. When his memory failed, they prescribed nootropics.

But the vampire knew. He tried to burn without fire. He tried to build without bone. And so, the vampire brought him marrow. The man cried as he ate it, because for the first time in years, he was not starving. He was being remembered.

His bloodwork told the same story his bones had been whispering: HDL in freefall. Triglycerides surging. Cortisol three times its baseline. His body was not thriving. It was surviving without fire.

The Metabolic Marriage

Protein without fat is incomplete nourishment. Fat provides fuel, regulates hormones, triggers satiety, carries fat-soluble vitamins (A, D, E, K), and converts into ketones: the brain's anti-inflammatory, anti-aging superfuel[1]. It also supplies **acetyl-CoA**, the critical entry molecule for the Krebs cycle. Excess protein burdens mitochondria with ammonia ... a metabolic tax that slows everything[2].

Without sufficient fat:

- Protein must be converted into glucose via gluconeogenesis, a taxing and inefficient backup process[3].
- Rabbit starvation, a condition seen in Arctic explorers who consumed only lean meat, can occur. Symptoms include nausea, fatigue, diarrhea, and eventual death[4].
- Vitamin deficiencies emerge. Without fat, the body cannot absorb vital nutrients needed for vision, bone health, immune function, and cellular repair[5].
- Vitamin K_2, found in grass-fed animal fats, is essential for directing calcium into bones and away from arteries. Its absence leads to calcification[6].
- Hormonal collapse ensues. Testosterone, estrogen, and progesterone are cholesterol-based. No fat means no fire for reproduction[7].
- Cholesterol also forms neurosteroids like allopregnanolone, crucial for brain resilience[8].

The kill was meant to warm you, not wear you down. And in every ancestral context, this truth was known:

- The Inuit discarded lean meat in times of famine, preferring fatty blubber[9].
- Native Americans mixed rendered fat with dried meat to make pemmican, a survival food with a 5:1 fat-to-protein ratio[10].
- The Hadza derive 50–70% of their calories from animal fat and discard lean game when abundance allows[11].
- Even lions leave the muscle if the organ-fat ratio is wrong. They prioritize marrow, organs, and visceral fat over pure muscle meat[12].

Fat and protein are biological partners, not enemies. You cannot burn one and ignore the other. You were built to eat both.

The Modern Dismemberment

Protein is everywhere now. In snack bars, yogurt pots, cereal, even water. High-protein. Low-fat. Guilt-free. The shelves are stocked with muscle, and stripped of marrow.

We've created a culture where protein is virtue and fat is vice. We praise 'lean meals', shame those who eat butter, glorify egg-white omelets while throwing away the yolk that carries the life-giving fat, choline, and vitamins[13].

Even gym culture clings to the myth that more protein equals more muscle. But studies show that hypertrophy plateaus beyond 1.6 grams per kilogram of body weight. More is not better[14].

Whey protein isolates, marketed as purity, strip away conjugated linoleic acid (CLA), milk fat phospholipids, and fat-soluble cofactors, turning nourishment into powder. The result? Inflammation, not information. We did not evolve this way.

- Our ancestors cracked bones for marrow.
- Ate liver first, not last.
- Gave fat to the elderly and children.

But now, we discard the fire. And then we shiver. To discard fat was to insult the spirit of the beast. The kill was only sacred when it was whole. They did not fear fat until they feared fertility. Until they feared their own hunger.

Spiritual Malnutrition

Without fat, the meal becomes performance, not communion. There is no satiety. No end. Only tracking macros on a screen, chewing skinless chicken while craving something nameless. The feast loses its wholeness.

Fat was never indulgent. It was sacred. It fed the brain, warmed the womb, built the child. It was the glow of the kill, the reward of risk, the taste of survival.

To discard it is to discard meaning. They tore the soul from the flesh, and called it clean. The vampire is not lean. He is not dry. He burns slow. Deep. On marrow and memory. The vampire watches. He knows that lean flesh without fat is not food. It is punishment. It is a body trying to survive without fire. But the fire remembers. And the fire returns.

Even the body remembers what modern menus forget. In women, body fat under 5% halts ovulation entirely. The womb shuts its gates. Fat was never excess. It was insurance… for life.

Reclaiming the Kill

To eat like a predator again:

- Choose cuts with visible fat.
- Eat the whole egg, not just the white.
- Render tallow and crack marrow bones
- Pair lean cuts with butter, yolk, or liver.
- Forget the macro calculator. Remember the kill.

You are not a spreadsheet. You are fire-bound flesh. Nature never served protein alone. She gave you flesh wrapped in flame. Eat both, or starve like the ones who forgot.

3.6 million years of hominin evolution never produced a 'low-fat' variant. Because without fat, there is no future.

Chapter 13

Sacred Blood, Forbidden Flesh

Where meat once made us holy, now it makes us guilty. This is no accident.

When Flesh Was a Prayer

We once ate in ceremony. Now we eat in shame. We offered the best. Now we hide the butcher. The altar has become the aisle.

Before calories had barcodes and cows had carbon scores, to eat meat was an act of devotion. Blood was not shameful; it was sacred. In every ancient culture that stared hunger in the eye and survived, the act of killing and eating was never taken lightly. Flesh was not fuel. It was covenant.

Picture a fire-lit altar in ancient Greece. The priests take the finest lamb, not the sick or the surplus, but the best. Its bones are wrapped in fat and burned, the smoke rising toward Olympus as an offering. The people eat only after the gods are fed. This was called *thysia*: a sacrifice to forge connection between heaven and hunger. Homer himself wrote that "the gods rejoiced in the savior of the feast."[1]

Meat wasn't mundane. It was myth. And in every myth, someone bleeds.

We did not eat blindly. We ate with awe. To chew was to cross a threshold. And the fire wasn't just for cooking; it was for consecration. A meal wasn't a macronutrient profile. It was a moment between mortality and the divine.

Kosher Cuts and the Right to Kill

In the Jewish tradition, that reverence becomes law. Not suggestion … law.

To eat meat, you must drain its blood. Not a drop remains. The *shechita*, the ritual slaughter, must be swift and clean, performed by a trained *shochet* using a flawless blade, and followed by a meticulous process of soaking and salting.[2]

Why? Because "the life of the flesh is in the blood," says Leviticus 17:11.[3] And life belongs to God. The blood must go back to the earth. To eat it would be to steal what was never yours.

It's not about bacteria. It's about boundaries. And about biology too: salting draws out iron and reduces oxidation, while preserving bioavailable zinc and vitamin B12.

The Torah doesn't forbid meat. It elevates it. In doing so, it demands accountability. You can eat, if you remember what was taken. The animal isn't a product. It's a life transferred, not consumed.

Each law is a tether. Each blessing, a reminder. Eating becomes an act of worship, and of restraint.

The vampire too obeys a code. He does not kill needlessly. He wastes nothing. He feeds with a reverence modern humans have forgotten.

The Lamb and the Ummah

In Islam, that reverence takes on communal form. Every year during Eid al-Adha, Muslims around the world commemorate Ibrahim's willingness to sacrifice his son by offering a lamb, or goat or cow, in his stead.

The animal is slaughtered by halal method: swift, intentional, and with the name of God on the tongue. A third of the meat is kept by the family, a third shared with relatives, and a third given to the poor.[4]

It is a sacred economy. Not of scarcity, but of structure. The meat is not devoured in private. It is distributed in the open, like blessing, like duty.

Where modern ideology avoids death, Islam ritualizes it. Where we sterilize the plate, they sanctify the knife. Not because they love blood, but because they understand its place.

The vampire understands this too. He does not hide his hunger. He honors it.

Blood for the Sun

Now shift your eyes west, to the high temples of Tenochtitlán. Here, the gods didn't want modesty. They wanted proof.

The Aztecs believed that the gods had sacrificed themselves to ignite the cosmos. Human blood, in turn, kept the sun moving. Huitzilopochtli, the sun god, demanded it daily.[5]

War captives were honored, not just punished, by being offered. Their hearts lifted to the sky, their bodies sometimes consumed in sacred feasts. The act was brutal. But it was also bound in reciprocity.

To modern eyes, it looks monstrous. But to the Aztecs, it was gratitude. It was continuity. The only way to avoid becoming prey to cosmic entropy was to feed the divine with flesh.

We recoil. But what is more barbaric: ceremonial sacrifice or industrial slaughter hidden behind glass and euphemism? Over 70 billion animals die each year in factories, nameless and unblessed. The Aztec priest knew the name of the life he ended.

The vampire, for all his myth, is more honest than the factory farm. He kills. But he knows why. And he remembers.

Cannibal God, Catholic Tongue

Christianity inherited the ritual, but flipped the altar. No more lambs. Now the god becomes the meat.

The Last Supper wasn't a metaphor picnic. "This is my body ... this is my blood" And then: eat. Catholic doctrine takes it seriously. Through transubstantiation, the bread becomes literal flesh. The wine, real blood.[6] It is tidy. Civilized. Clean. No blood on the altar, only gold chalices hiding the metaphor's iron truth.

But underneath lies something older and deeper: the idea that communion only comes through consumption. That we must integrate the divine through mouth and gut. That flesh is knowledge. And science now whispers the same. Peptides like carnosine in red meat cross the blood-brain barrier, altering neurochemistry for clarity and resolve.

The vampire knows this by instinct. He drinks to live, but he also drinks to know. Blood carries memory. Lineage. Spirit.

So does steak. You just forgot.

The Woman Who Cooked in Silence

She never prayed aloud. Not anymore. There had once been blessings in her mother's kitchen. Incantations whispered as the onions hit the pan. Bones kissed with vinegar and fire. The meat was salted with memory. Rituals handed down, not written, but remembered.

But the world changed. Supermarkets replaced smoke. Microwave hums replaced firelight. Her daughter learned about food from cartoons and dietary guidelines. The family table, once carved from wood and waiting, was now cluttered with devices and plastic wrappers.

So she cooked in silence. The lamb's heart she sourced from the backroom butcher. The liver, she cleaned with vinegar and citrus, just like her grandmother had. She set the table with care, real plates, real knives, no packets in sight.

And when the meal was ready, she didn't speak. She just placed the heart at the center of the table, the bone broth beside it, the roasted marrow in a small, sacred dish.

Her daughter stared. "Where's the sauce?" She replied, "This is the sauce." The marrow glistened like liquid amber. The broth steamed like temple incense.

She watched as her child, slowly, took the first bite. The room was still. Something ancient stirred.

Afterward, the girl said nothing, but she helped clean up. Carefully. She handled the bones like heirlooms. She asked, softly, what part of the lamb the marrow came from. And when the next meal came, she brought salt to the table without being asked.

The woman never said a word. But the blessing had returned. And in her heart, she whispered what her grandmother once whispered: *Tȟatȟáŋka čhaŋté čik'ala.* (Buffalo heart makes our hearts strong.)

Meat, Memory, and the Maternal Flame

In almost every ancestral culture, women were not just firekeepers. They were memory keepers. They preserved recipes, but more than that, they preserved rituals. They knew which parts of the animal to save for healing, which fats to feed the children, and how to honor the kill with flavor, story, and salt.

In Lakota tradition, women butchered the bison with prayers for each organ: "The heart for courage, the tongue for truth, the liver for vision." Fat was rendered into pȟežúta sápa, "black medicine," used to heal wounds and seal covenants.[7] When colonizers slaughtered the herds, they didn't just starve bodies. They severed a sacred female lineage where every cut was liturgy.

Even the Vestals guarded the flame that turned flesh to sacrament. Without fire, meat was just rotting carrion.[8]

The kitchen was never just domestic. It was sacred. To prepare meat was to remember death, and to serve it was to pass on strength. And when we erased these rituals, we didn't just forget nutrition. We forgot reverence.

Philosophy in the Fat

Modern people have inherited a crisis: we want meaning without mess. We want to be sacred and sanitary. We want life without death. Nutrition without nature. So we invent substitutes: soy-based, pea-protein, sterile, lab-grown.

We worship the corpse of food, embalmed in plastic and called virtue. The less life it cost, the more praise it earns.

We slap "humane certified" stickers on vacuum-packed guilt. We pay carbon offsets like medieval indulgences, buying absolution for the sin of consumption. The factory cow dies alone, unnamed, unmourned. But we feel virtuous because the package says "grass-fed." This isn't ethics. It's atonement theatre.

Today, 84% of Americans say they feel no connection to the source of their food. But her daughter brought the salt without being asked.

The Aztec priest knew the cost of his knife. We outsource ours to slaughterhouses and feel clean. But without sacrifice, the meal means nothing. We do not bless our food. We scan it. We do not thank the animal. We fear the fat.

Food has never been morally neutral. It has always been a spiritual act. It reveals who we are, what we revere, and what we fear. To eat blood is to affirm the cycle. To eat fat is to accept our own need. To eat meat is to remember that something dies so that something else may thrive. The vampire is not a monster. He is a mirror. He doesn't represent death. He represents memory of it.

Lucien's Prayer

Some vampires hunt with lust. But Lucien, the oldest I knew, hunted with reverence. Before feeding, he'd press his palm to the victim's forehead, not to hypnotize, but to honor. "I take your life so I may live," he'd whisper. "Your breath becomes my memory."

Modern humans consume lifeless protein shakes. Vampires consume legacy. The difference isn't in the blood. It's in the blessing.

One night, Lucien sampled beef from a supermarket tray. He chewed, then stilled. "This blood remembers nothing," he said. And did not finish the meal.

Vampires Don't Apologize

And neither should you.

The vampire remembers. The shepherd remembers. The mother who cooked in silence remembers. The priest, the warrior, the hunter, the child, they all once knew this truth: That meat is more than matter. That fat is not shame; it's surplus made sacred. That blood is remembrance.

You are not a sinner for eating. You are not a monster for hungering. You are a creature of ritual, born in blood and lit by fire. Reclaim the knife stained with truth and terra cotta. Reclaim the fire that consecrates the feast. And eat like something sacred still burns in you

Chapter 14

The Nightshade and the Nightmare

Nature is not benevolent. It is efficient.

A Tale of Toxic Salads, Stealthy Plants, and the Botany of Betrayal

Once upon a time, in the soft-lit aisles of Whole Foods, a shopper gazed lovingly at a plump eggplant, unaware she was cradling a botanical booby trap. She would later bake it with turmeric, quinoa, and righteousness, then post the recipe with hashtags about healing and gut health. Two hours later, she'd be bloated, fatigued, and mildly irritated with her husband for no discernible reason. And yet she'd do it again. Why? Because plants, dear reader, are not your friends.

Contrary to every broccoli-wielding nutritionist with a food pyramid tattoo, the green things on your plate do not exist to nourish you. They exist to survive you.

This chapter is an exorcism. A heresy. A toxic take on toxic plants. It's where we peel back the chlorophyll smile and expose the nightmare in the nightshade. Because behind every 'superfood' lurks a supervillain.

The Botanical Conspiracy

It's time we had a difficult conversation about kale. And spinach. And that smug little almond in your oat-free granola.

We have been trained to view plants as passive providers, generous green givers of life. Their leaves, fruits, seeds, and roots are portrayed as offerings, freely given for the benefit of human health and digestive enlightenment. This narrative works beautifully. Except for one minor detail: plants do not want to be eaten.

Unlike animals, which can run, bite, kick, or moo plaintively when threatened, plants had to invent another strategy for survival. And so they turned to chemistry. The evolutionary arms race between herbivore and herb is older than language itself. The battlefield is biochemical. Plants developed:

- Oxalates, which bind calcium, cause kidney stones, and irritate tissues
- Lectins, which pierce the gut lining and trigger immune dysfunction
- Phytates, which block mineral absorption like dietary bouncers
- Saponins, which foam and puncture intestinal wall
- Glucosinolates, which break down into goitrogens and disrupt thyroid function

In short, plants are not passive. They are biochemical saboteurs. Ignore their tricks at your peril.

Yes, human bodies co-evolved defenses: liver enzymes; gut flora; bile salts; mucin layers; and detox enzymes. But those defenses evolved for seasonal nibbles, not daily kale smoothies and oxalate boosters. We were never meant to ingest this kind of chronic phytochemical load.

Nightshades and Other Demons

Enter the nightshades, the goths of the vegetable world. Tomatoes, potatoes, eggplants, peppers - members of the Solanaceae family. Their appeal is Mediterranean. Their effect is medieval.

Nightshades contain alkaloids like solanine and nicotine. These might be entertaining in a Victorian opium den but are less welcome in your salad. A single green potato can harbor 100 mg of solanine[1], enough to cause nausea, hallucinations, paralysis, or a bad poetry reading. While toxicity typically requires a higher dose (20–40 mg/kg body weight[2]), even low doses may provoke inflammation in susceptible individuals.

Solanine lurks in tomato stems, green peppers, and eggplant skins. It is nature's insurance policy against overeating. These compounds are neurotoxic in sufficient quantities and inflammatory in far smaller ones. They sneak past your gut lining, tripwire your immune system, and often trigger symptoms in joints, skin, and cognition.

Ask the autoimmune crowd. The connection between "clean eating" and flaring symptoms is not anecdotal; it is biochemical[3]. Inflammatory bowel conditions, eczema, arthritis, chronic fatigue... all can be amplified by the very foods we're told to worship.

For genetically susceptible individuals, such as those who carry the HLA-B27 gene variant[4], nightshades can be landmines. While most people tolerate them, these individuals may suffer flares that don't read nutrition labels.

And spinach? It's practically a crystal meth lab for oxalates[5]. That green smoothie might look like health, but it stings like oxalic acid in your bladder.

The Salad Illusion

There is a peculiar moral purity surrounding plant-based diets. Leaf-eating is treated not just as smart, but as virtuous. A kind of nutritional sainthood conferred by crunching raw foliage in open-plan offices. But dig beneath the compost and you'll find something darker.

The raw vegan is a modern-day monk. Their pain is part of the performance. Bloating is a baptism. Gas is growth. Faintness? A spiritual fast-track. They do not eat to nourish; they eat to atone. Salads are our era's hair shirt.

We've moralized the plant. Wrapped it in ecology, ethics, and enlightenment. But plants don't reciprocate. They don't reward us for our virtue. They punish indiscriminately. And so we find ourselves in a strange position: inflamed, deficient, yet spiritually smug.

Meanwhile, the corporate wellness machine packages your suffering and sells it back to you as enlightenment. Oxalate-laden "superfood" powders are marketed to detox you, while silently leaching calcium from your bones. A whole industry profits from your micronutrient malabsorption. It's dietary Stockholm syndrome with more Tupperware.

Ancestral Eating: We Knew Better

Here's the punchline. Your ancestors already figured this out. For millennia, humans treated plants with suspicion and respect. Bitter leaves were avoided unless cooked, soaked, fermented, or pounded into submission. Tribes knew which tubers to detoxify in streams, which mushrooms to fear, and which seeds to crush before consumption. This wasn't superstition. It was survival.

Different cultures adapted with different detox strategies. Indigenous Americans nixtamalized corn. Africans fermented cassava. Siberians soaked wild potatoes in ash. You, however, toss raw kale into a blender and hashtag #cleaneating while your thyroid stages a mutiny. (Which, for the record, cooking and adequate iodine intake can often prevent[6].)

Fermentation, slow-cooking, and even ash-soaking weren't rituals. They were anti-nutrient mitigation strategies. You think soaking beans is about softness? No. It's about not dying.

Modern agriculture, meanwhile, has bred many of these same plants to be sweeter and prettier, but not less toxic. The bitterness may be gone, but the biochemistry still bites. Oxalate content in spinach, for example, has risen over 300% since 1950[7].

Your great-grandmother fermented cabbage. You social-media #livingfoods and pay the price.

The Garden That Bit Back

In the green shadow of a forgotten village, there lived a man named Elias who grew the most splendid vegetables. His garden teemed with life. Leaves unfurled like scrolls. Fruits glistened with promise.

One day, he discovered a vine he didn't recognize. It bore crimson pods shaped like hearts. Curious and proud, Elias tasted one. It burned his tongue and made his vision shimmer. That night, he dreamed of roots wrapping around his bedpost.

In the weeks that followed, Elias changed. He grew pale and jittery. His joints cracked like twigs in the cold. He lost weight but swore he had never felt "cleaner." He began sleeping in the soil. Said the earth whispered recipes. His neighbors avoided him, unnerved by the strange hum in the hedgerows and the way flies lingered on his breath.

When they found him months later, he was naked among the leaves. His eyes were glassy, skin inflamed, fingernails black. The pods were everywhere. None of them dared touch them. But the pods pulsed softly in the moonlight, whispering: "Eat clean. Suffer quietly. Post your plate."

Note: Elias's fate isn't pure fiction. Case reports have documented oxalate nephropathy in 'green smoothie cleansers'[8]... real-life versions of the garden that bit back.

Moral of the Meal

This is not a crusade against plants. It is a call to reframe them. Plants are not benign. They are chemically armed negotiators with their own agendas. They can heal, harm, and hinder - often in the same meal. Respecting them means not being seduced by their Instagram filters.

Most demand respect, not reverence. Boil the bitterness to submission. Cook them. Ferment them. Neutralize their traps. Or, for best results, simply eat fewer of them.

Because meat never hid its nature. Blood, bone, and brutal honesty. It didn't pretend to be light and love. It didn't have a lectin problem. It didn't sting your kidneys. It fed your ancestors with muscle and marrow.

The true betrayal was not in eating meat. It was in trading it for a green dream wrapped in inflammation.

The druid was poisoned, but wise. Nature isn't benevolent. But with ancestral wisdom, it can be bargained with.

Chapter 15

The Pulse of Death

They gave up lions for lentils. But the hunger never left.

The Taste of Surrender

No empire is built on steak. It may be won by men who eat it, but it is maintained with mush. With porridge. With barley paste. With lentil stew, ladled out with institutional indifference and a side of moral rhetoric.

Grain is the great pacifier, a muzzle for the human spirit. It fills the belly but dulls the instinct. It nourishes the flesh just enough to keep it docile. It replaces the fire in the gut with a gurgle.

There's a reason the vampire doesn't eat soup. He fasts between kills. He feeds on vitality. He drinks blood, not broth. The predator is not always eating. But when he does, it matters. The vampire is ancestral wisdom, unapologetic, nutrient-focused, and distrustful of mush.

The modern citizen? Snack-fed, soy-lulled, spreadsheet-compliant. A eunuch of appetite.

Vampires don't eat porridge. Neither should you.

Cain Kills, Abel Farms

The first meal worth killing for was meat. Cain tilled the soil. Abel kept flocks. Cain offered grains. Abel offered meat. God chose Abel. So, Cain killed his brother.

It was more than a murder. It was a rebellion. A farmer's revolt against the sacred order of blood. Cain wanted his crops to be enough. Abel knew they never could be. Cain's curse echoes in every lab-grown burger and lentil-loaf sermon. We are all sons of Cain now. But some of us remember.

Some say Cain's descendants buried the Boneknife, the blade forged from the rib of the First Beast. Some say it still whispers in dark corners of the earth... especially when lentils boil.

Some say Garron's blood still runs in those who refuse the spoon.

Science in the Stew

Now for the quiet facts beneath the fire. Lentils contain:

- Lectins, which can damage intestinal lining.
- Phytic acid, which inhibits zinc, iron, and calcium absorption.
- Oxalates, which contribute to kidney stones.

Traditional processing reduces lectins and phytates but never eliminates them[1]. Fermentation mitigates some harms, but never replaces the hunt. They lack:

- B12
- Heme iron
- Creatine
- Preformed Vitamin A (retinol)
- Long-chain Omega-3s (DHA)
- Cholesterol (precursor to sex hormones)

In contrast, meat provides these nutrients in dense, bioavailable form[2] [3]. Your mitochondria don't care about ethics. They want nutrients. And lentils don't deliver.

Of Monks and Monsters

The monk eats lentils. The vampire eats meat. One fasts to flee desire. The other fasts to sharpen it. One sterilizes instinct. The other exalts it. One eats to survive. The other eats to remember.

The monk chants. The vampire stalks. The monk shrinks. The vampire endures. The monk spreadsheets fasts. The vampire spreadsheets hunts.

This is not moral judgment. It's metabolic realism.

The monk sacrifices his hunger on the altar of control. The vampire feeds only when the world forgets its fear. One is praised. The other, punished.

But the vampire never apologizes for his appetite. Why should you? Vampires don't eat porridge. And they don't count calories.

A Brief History of Grain-Based Control

Let us now turn to history, not for nostalgia, but for truth.

Agriculture traded biological vitality for caloric security. A Faustian bargain that birthed empires but shrank skeletons.

In ancient Babylon, temple workers were paid in beer and barley. This was not charity. It was chess. Feed the worker just enough to work. Never enough to revolt[4].

In Rome, plebeians were pacified with *annona*: monthly wheat rations that became bread, then dependence, then silence. Two hundred thousand mouths fed not to strengthen the people, but to still them[5].

In colonial India and Africa, the British replaced meat-rich traditional diets with pulses and grains. It was not nutrition. It was governance. "Relief efforts" introduced lentils not to restore life, but to manage it[6].

Hunters remember autonomy. Gruel-eaters forget. The ruling class dined on flesh. The workers, on mush. History whispers: lentils tame lions. Biology roars back.

The Pulse of Empire

Behold the lentil. Small. Bland. Virtue-flavored. It does not roar or rot or run. It stores forever. It cooks to mush. It demands no death, no blade, no memory. It is the food of bureaucrats. Of monks. Of spreadsheets and slogans.

You can grow millions of them. You can package them with a smile. You can pair them with carbon offsets and infographics. You can serve them to a nation and call it progress. But no warrior dreams of lentils. The lentil is not a meal. It's a moral performance.

The King Who Fed Them Lentils

There was once a king who ruled a fierce land, where the people lived on blood and fire. Hunters. Warriors. Children of meat and bone. But the king grew weary of rebellion. He wanted peace. And peace, he knew, came not from strength, but from softness. So, he banned the hunt. He outlawed the fire. He built kitchens that served only lentils.

At first, the people resisted. So, he made the lentils symbolic. "They are a gesture of compassion," he said. "A balm for the Earth." He paid poets to write odes to legumes. He promoted dietitians to prophets. He declared chewing jerky a sin against the state.

And slowly, the fire dimmed. The men lost their edge. The women their moonblood[10]. The children, their wild eyes. Until one day, a child asked: "Why do we eat mush?"

The child's question hung unanswered. For the language of fire had been lost, replaced by the whisper of spoons.

If you want to tame a lion, don't chain it. Feed it lentils.

Modern Mush: From Rome to the UN

Today, the Roman dole lives on in new robes.

- UN programs prioritize grains and pulses (cost efficiency is greater than nutrition)[8].
- School lunches exalt tofu over liver.
- The EAT-Lancet Commission's "Planetary Health Diet" recommends mostly legumes, with meat limited to 14g daily[7] (a sacrament, not a meal).

These efforts are often born from good intentions - to feed the hungry, to stabilize communities, to serve the many. But the outcome betrays the biology. The compassion becomes compliance. The nutrition becomes narrative. The "Planetary Health Diet" sacrifices human biology for spreadsheet ecology. Silvopasture and regenerative grazing nourish soil where lentils deplete it.

Meanwhile:

- Obesity climbs.
- Testosterone plummets.
- Fertility shrinks (sperm counts halved since 1973[9]... and amplified by plastics, stress, and endocrine disruptors).

- Children chew glyphosate-dusted pseudo meat shaped like extinct beasts and wonder why they feel anxious.

Lentils feed ledgers. Meat feeds lineages.

How to Spot a Nutritional Lie (It usually has a label)

- It speaks in 'health claims' but never in hunger.
- It praises moral restraint but punishes biological truth.
- It comes with an environmental sermon and a celebrity chef.
- It never bleeds.
- It doesn't rot.
- It avoids ancestral foods and embraces patented ones.
- It asks you to trust the science - just not your body.
- Follow the money: $100 million buys a lot of tofu sermons.

Food was once a story of fire, not a spreadsheet. If it needs a label, it probably forgot the knife.

The Night the Lentils Burned

The temple kitchens had burned before anyone realized they were flammable. For fifty years, they had simmered nothing but lentil mush. No fat. No fire. Just policy. Porridge. Peace.

Then came Garron. He brought no manifesto. Only fat. Flame. Ancestral rage. By morning, smoke curled over the hills. Ash coated the sacred gardens. In the ruins, searchers found no monks - only bones. Goat bones. Pig bones. Cow bones. And one thing more: A knife. Carved from bone. Ancient. Still sharp.

Some said it was the same blade Mira once wielded. The Boneknife. Hidden. Preserved. Waiting. The fire had unveiled what the doctrine had buried. This had once been a place of sacrifice. Of meat. Of flame. Before the Lentil Mandate. Before the Great Tranquility. Before compliance became gospel.

That winter, wild pigs returned to the hills. Children learned to trap again. And Garron disappeared. Vanished into myth, or mist, or memory.

A stew without death is just starch. A life without fire is just existence.

The Ox and the Lion

In ancient bestiaries, two archetypes ruled: The ox: yoked, obedient, herbivorous. The lion: wild, proud, carnivorous. The ox is bred to serve. The lion lives on instinct.

Modern culture worships the ox. Work hard. Chew quietly. Don't question the feed. But the vampire remembers the lion. And so should you. Choose the lion's iron. Spit out the ox's yoke.

Chapter 16

The Eternal Meal - Feasting, Fasting, and the Cycles of the Wild

In the wild, hunger is not a flaw. It is the beginning of memory.

You were never meant to graze. You were meant to feast and fast, To kill, then wait. To starve, then rise.

Modern hunger is not hunger. It is interference. A synthetic rhythm imposed by convenience, softened by snacks, numbed by schedule. The real hunger, the wild hunger, was sacred. It stalked. It struck. It sanctified the body with fire. That cycle was not broken. It was buried.

The Clock That Forgot the Kill

'Three meals a day' is not a biological truth. It's an industrial spell. It wasn't carved into bone. It was printed on factory walls.

Before the bell, before the boxed lunch, before the portable snack, there was the kill. The body knew only feast and famine. Hunting meant absence. Eating meant ceremony. Nothing in nature eats at intervals. Everything eats in response. The nine-to-five meal schedule is a cage for predators. Lions eat when the prey is down, not when a bell rings. Why don't you?

The Lunar Table

Ancient calendars didn't track time in hours. They tracked it in hunger.

Ramadan's sunup-fast and sundown-feast mirror the hunter's return. Lent's forty-day abstention echoes winter scarcity before spring's kill. The Day of Atonement in Judaism binds the body to the moon's hunger cycle[1]. Even pagan solstice rites followed the tilt of the Earth's appetite. So did agricultural fasts like the Eleusinian Mysteries, voluntary abstention amid abundance.

Centuries before labs, these rites knew: Fasting sharpens cognition and kindles cellular repair[10]. Your mitochondria still hum with ancient hunger. You didn't always eat. Because there wasn't always food. And when you did eat, it was not in shame. It was in ceremony.

The Hunger That Hunted

Every predator obeys the cycle: stalk, kill, feast, fast. This isn't philosophy. It's physiology. Fasting is not starvation. It is signal. It is precision. It sharpens the eye. It prepares the strike.

The Hadza of Tanzania do not graze. They hunt. They dig. They endure. When the hunt fails, they wait. Not by choice, but by design[3]. They may taste honey or baobab along the way, but the feast is earned, not scheduled.

These fasts are not virtuous. They are visceral. Unplanned. Unapologetic. Nature doesn't grant participation medals. It grants only the kill, or the wait. Hunger isn't an alarm to silence. It's a compass to follow.

The Hormones That Remember

Hunger isn't a flaw. It's a message. Ghrelin rises like a hunter's call, not with panic, but with purpose[4]. It sharpens focus, not just appetite. Eat breakfast daily at 8 a.m., and ghrelin will show up on time, every time. But that's entrainment, not instinct.

True hunger builds with silence, not with routine. And when the feast comes? Leptin from steak whispers satisfaction. Leptin from cereal screams more.

At night, melatonin rises, insulin drops, and the cells clean house. This is circadian autophagy[5], the nightly ritual of renewal. Disrupt that, and you don't just lose sleep. You lose memory. You lose rhythm. Blue light at night sedates the fire. It steals melatonin, disrupts autophagy, and rewrites the rhythm. You chew not from hunger, but from stress. Cortisol in disguise.

The female body listens to moon and cycle. Follicular fasting is fire. Luteal phases may ask for fuel.

The False Feast

Cereal at dawn. Snack bar at ten. Shake at noon. Pasta at midnight. A drip-feed of forgetting. You are not nourished. You are sedated. There is no feast. There is no famine. There is only the interruptive chew of fear.

You don't need more food. You need more rhythm. You don't need more calories. You need more memory.

The Woman Who Waited

There was a woman named Sil. She believed hunger meant failure. That missing meals meant collapse. She drank green sludge and counted almonds. Her hands trembled. Her brain fogged. Hashimoto's, they said. Fatigue. Pills.

But before the diagnosis, she'd had a dream. Of scrolls wrapped in bone. Of a fire carved into stone. Of words that pulsed like memory: "In the wild, hunger is not a flaw. It is the beginning of memory."

Then came her refusal. Twelve hours. Then sixteen. Then twenty. The hunger came. But so did the vision. Her antibodies halved, not from pills, but from three blood-moons of fasting[10]. She fasted like a lioness. She feasted like a warrior. She never chewed in fear again.

The cure isn't in the calendar. It's in the kill.

The Man Who Found the Flame

He was efficient. Tracked macros. Avoided hunger. Until his father died, full of pills and soup. The grief didn't break him. The flavorless sandwich did.

Two days passed. He didn't eat. Didn't mean to. On the third, in the woods, he smelled fire. Not smoke. Fire. Mira's color, blood-orange and bone-white. He took venison. He lit the flame. He fed the silence.

Now he fasts every full moon. Hunts alone. Feeds with fire. And lives. Hunger is the doorway. Fire is the guide. Flesh is the return.

The Feastfire Rite

In the valley where the red moon rose, the people fasted for three days. Only broth. Only silence.

Then came the fire. Then came the kill. One animal. One blaze. One meal. They called it the Feastfire Rite. As with the Inuit *Aiviq* whale feast, hunger made the flame sacred. Until a leader outlawed the fast. Declared it "cruel." Declared crops superior. Built storage. Served starch.

"Why suffer?" he asked. "Let there be daily meals."

And so, there were. The fire dimmed. The children softened. The stories stopped. He died swollen on starch, fat, forgotten, full of nothing.

Then a child rose. Whispered "For Mira." Disappeared into the forest. Returned with a boar. Lit the fire herself. No permission. No priest. Just flame. And memory.

A culture that forgets feasting forgets who it is.

The Metabolic Pulse

Fasting activates:

- Autophagy, peaking at 24–48 hours[6]
- Ketones, the brain's ancestral fuel[7]
- Growth hormone, surging for repair[8-9]
- Insulin sensitivity, renewed
- Testosterone, rising acutely in fasted states[9] (prolonged may lower[11])
- Cellular memory, sharpened

Feasting restores:

- Leptin
- Thyroid hormones
- Bone growth
- Creatine, cholesterol, B12
- Glycogen (muscle fuel)
- Ritual. Rhythm. Reverence.

This isn't a trick. It's a return. Your ancestors didn't fear emptiness. They used it.

Vampires Feast at Midnight

I do not sip broth at board meetings. I do not nibble compliance. I fast because it teaches. I feast because it remembers. I've hunted beneath eclipses. Lit flame beneath the Feastfire stones. Drunk the blood of beasts and kin. Tracked blood-moons, not time zones.

Like predators who feast at dusk or dawn, not under fluorescent glare, I remember when humans lit solstice fires, not midnight snacks. And I do not apologize. You can keep grazing. Or you can wake up.

Note to the Reader

The next time you feel the ache, the honest ache of hunger, wait. Not to punish. But to prepare. Light fire. Hunt memory. Eat flesh. Not like a clock. But like a wolf who sees the moon.

You are not broken for waiting. You are a creature of rhythm. Of silence and flame.

Fasting Framework

- **Circadian fasting**: 13-16 hours - best for daily metabolic reset
- **Lunar fasting**: 24-48 hours - supports autophagy and cellular repair
- **Seasonal fasting**: 3-7 days - allows immune recalibration

Chapter 17

The Mirror of Meat - Flesh, Shame, and the Blood Beneath the Skin

When people eat meat, they change. They stop nibbling and start hunting.

You were not born ashamed of meat. You were taught that shame. Taught to see steak as sin. Taught to see muscle as threat. Taught to whisper "sorry" every time your body begged for blood.

Meat is no longer just meat. It is metaphor. It is motive. It is charged, gendered, politicized, and weaponized. A ribeye is now a Rorschach test: project shame or sovereignty. Masculinity? Caricatured. Femininity? Fluid. And meat? Dangerous.

They say it pollutes the planet, fuels aggression, breeds violence. But beneath these claims lies something deeper... an unease with flesh itself. An anxiety about strength. A fear of appetite.

We have made meat taboo because we have made power taboo. And behind that taboo, we forgot a truth. You were not born with a tag in your ear and a schedule in your mouth. You were born wild, and wild things eat flesh.

The Flame Beneath Gender

Across time, meat was not male, it was sacred.

Achilles feasted before battle. Ishtar received bull's flesh in blood rites. In Norse myth, the gods ate boar every night to maintain their vitality before the end of the world. In these myths, flesh was not dominance. It was divine restoration.

Yet today, red meat is framed as hypermasculine. As a relic of the caveman. A fossil of testosterone-fueled tyranny. This is not science. It is social engineering. Because in the body, meat does not discriminate.

Without dietary cholesterol, women's hormone synthesis falters.[1] Without heme iron, pregnancy becomes risk.[2] B12 deficiency affects cognition in all sexes.[3] Women on low-meat diets have a 50% higher risk of amenorrhea.[13] Men on vegan diets show testosterone levels 30% lower than omnivores.[14] Protein and fat are the scaffolds of life, not political mascots.

To eat meat is not to oppress. It is to obey your design. True masculinity was never about domination. It was about direction, strength channeled into service. The predator as protector. The firebearer, not the bully.

The Fat-Soluble Truth

Vitamins A, D, E, and K2, the great fat-soluble quartet, do not thrive in spinach. They live in liver, butter, egg yolks, and bone marrow.[4] They shape the immune system, the brain, the bones. Vitamin K2 puts calcium where it belongs: into the skeleton, not the arteries.[5] Vitamin A lights the skin and the night-vision of warriors. Vitamin D orchestrates hormones.

Without cholesterol, your body cannot make pregnenolone, without pregnenolone, none of these essential hormones such as progesterone, testosterone, and aldosterone can exist. No bypass, no shortcut, no hormones.[1] Tryptophan and tyrosine, precursors to serotonin and dopamine, come not from chickpeas but from steak.[6]

To eat meat is not to signal aggression. It is to give the brain what it needs to feel joy.

The Butcher's Daughter

The man was crying in her chair again. Every Tuesday, 4:10 p.m. Lavender cologne. Apologetic eyes. Same order... a bone-in ribeye, thick as shame.

She wrapped it in butcher's paper, her father's Boneknife gleaming under glass. "I'm sorry," he whispered, "I know it's bad for..."

She held up a bloodstained hand. "My father said guilt ruins the meat." He blinked. "Sorry?" "You chew it. Swallow it. Then lie about how good it was. That's not virtue. That's cowardice."

The next week he didn't come. Nor the next. But on the third, he returned. No apology. Just hunger. She smiled. "Good. Now let's feed something real."

Feminine Hunger

It's not just men who've been shamed. The war on meat has wounded women too, but more quietly. For centuries, red meat was part of the feminine rite. Women bled, and then they ate. Liver was prized. Fat was sacred.

Fertility was fed, not feared. Grandmothers served tongue and bone marrow to postpartum daughters. There was no shame in animal hunger. There was only reverence for strength.

But in the 20th century, something changed. Meat became 'heavy.' 'Manly.' 'Gross.' Women were encouraged to eat salads, not steaks. To avoid cholesterol. To fear fat. To shrink. So, they did. Iron levels dropped.[7] Energy declined. Fertility rates fell.[8] Ovaries went quiet.

But the ads kept coming, telling women they were empowered… so long as they stayed light, tame, and meatless. The hunger didn't go away. It just got dressed in yoga pants, drowned in oat milk and hashtags. Salads build virtue. Steak builds life.

The Forgotten Goddesses

They said Lilith left Eden because she refused to submit. But what they didn't say is what she ate. She found blood in the wilderness. Killed a bird with her hands. Drank from bone. Sank her teeth into raw liver. And something in her changed. Not monstrous, mammalian. Not wicked, awake.

Artemis, too, lived outside the garden. Bow in hand. Boar on her back. The moon at her feet. Her arrow was carved from the same bone as Mira's knife. She fed on fat and hunted without apology. These were not goddesses of submission. They were women of instinct. And every bite of flesh was a spell cast against domestication.

Lilith's fire burned in Mira's hands, and now yours.

The Culture War on Carnivores

You were told that eating meat made you violent. Or worse, unfashionable. You saw magazine covers celebrate plant-based purity: thin limbs, soft bellies, moral halos. You heard celebrities declare they had 'transcended' flesh. You watched documentaries show athletes 'powered by plants,' only to learn later they'd gone back to eggs and fish when the cameras stopped rolling.[9] This isn't science. It's theatre.

The war on meat is a war on vitality. A war on autonomy. A war on remembering what nourishes you. Because when people eat meat, they change. They stand taller. Think clearer. Speak louder. They say "no" more often. They trade forks for fangs. They remember the Boneknife. And systems of control do not like that.

The Husband Who Hid

Every night, he waited until she slept. He'd open the back door. Step into the garage. And pull from behind the freezer a Tupperware marked "cauliflower." Inside was bacon. Cold. Cooked in secret. He didn't tell her. Didn't tell anyone. Just chewed in the dark like a guilty animal. His cholesterol was fine. His shame was not.

Then one day, she found him mid-bite. Said nothing. Just stared. He swallowed. "I miss it," he said. "I miss feeling like a man." She nodded. The next night, she joined him. Two steaks. Two mouths. No shame.

The System's Soft Weapon

Hollywood sells two kinds of men: the soy-soft hero or the psychotic carnivore. Marvel's quinoa-chewing Thor replaced Norse mythology's boar-devouring Odin.

In wellness circles, women are applauded for eating less, juicing more, and starving in the name of balance. Meanwhile, "sustainable" brands push cricket protein and lab-grown pseudo flesh as progressive. This is not about food. It's about compliance.

When a people are well-fed, they question. When a people are weak, they obey. Meat doesn't just nourish muscle. It nourishes muscle and moral courage.[12]

A woman who eats liver is harder to manipulate. A man who eats steak is harder to shame. A child raised on marrow laughs at propaganda. This isn't a diet. It's a quiet rebellion.

The Inclusive Flame

Modern gender narratives twist nourishment into performance. Men are told to be softer: less primal, less hungry, less 'problematic.' Women are told to be lighter: less dense, less demanding, less bloody. So both shrink. Shrink their portions. Shrink their instincts. Shrink their fire.

But the body cannot be fooled forever. Low-fat diets do not build ovaries. Soy silences ovulation.[10] Liver restores it. Soy milk does not menstruate. It mimics. It masks. But it does not nourish. You are flesh. You require flesh. Not just for muscle or mitochondria, but for memory.

Meat shame targets all who defy 'acceptable' hunger - gentle men, butch women, and those outside binaries. Flesh liberates every body.

The Inuit knew: 'Fat is life.' Modern diets call it suicide.[11]

The Vampire Remembers

You were not shamed by meat until they taught you to chew without pride. You were not afraid of flesh until they wrapped it in sin. You were not broken until they told you your hunger was. You were not lost until you stopped listening to your blood.

Meat is not a show. It is a mirror. It reveals your relationship to hunger. To power. To shame. It asks: Do you consume with reverence, or apology? Do you hide your instincts, or honor them? In this mirror, you do not see ideology. You see identity.

The vampire watches. The vampire waits. And when he feeds, it is not performance. It is presence. The vampire's reflection shows no ideology, only the bones of your hunger. Flesh was never the enemy. Flesh was the truth.

I have seen empires fall when men forgot liver and women feared blood. I have seen centuries pass like shadows. I have watched queens faint from salad. I have watched kings apologize for teeth. I have seen hunger repackaged as 'discipline,' and satiety punished as sin.

But... I never knelt to salad. I have fasted under comets. Feasted in ice. Bled in deserts. And every time I chewed flesh, I remembered... I was not made to be harmless. I was made to be honest. So now I ask you. Will you keep grazing, guilt-wracked and gelded from your power? Or will you bite?

There is no virtue in weakness. No wisdom in apology. Only the steady, roaring truth of blood, fat, and fire.

Look into the mirror. Sink your teeth into what they forbade. Become what you were. Eat like the flame remembers or starve like the system demands.

The mirror remembers. And now... so do you!

Chapter 18

The Cold-Blooded Ritual - Fasting, Frost, and the Forge Within

Cold is not absence. It is fire sleeping, waiting for hunger to wake it.

Predator Tempered

A well-fed man is a slow man. Softness is a comfort blanket soaked in decay. Your ancestors knew the ritual. Strip the warmth. Delay the feast. Let sensation sharpen. Let suffering sculpt. A predator does not prepare with comfort. He prepares with pain.

I was forged in fire, quenched in ice.

Season of Teeth

Winter was not a threat. It was the season of teeth. Before thermostats, the Sámi drank reindeer blood on ice. The Inuit ate frozen whale blubber raw.

Sámi herders showed twelve-degree lower shivering thresholds than urban Swedes[9]. Inuit hunters metabolized seal fat at minus thirty with stable core temperatures[10].

They didn't just endure cold, they weaponized it. Frostbite was not failure... it was initiation. When skin blackened, the elders whispered: "Now you begin to live." They became wolves of frost and famine.

Ice and Ember

Fasting is the fast. Cold is the blade. One clears the path, the other sharpens the edge.

Fasting strips the buffer. Cold strips the illusion. Both tear away the veil that comfort drapes over your instincts. Together, they sculpt the body, mind and myth.

Threshold Twins - Fasting and Cold as Sacred Gates

Fasting and cold are not cousins. They are twins, born of the same icy womb. Both demand you cross a threshold: Fasting, the gasp when glycogen fades and ketones rise; Cold, the burn when skin screams and brown fat ignites. Both trigger the same ancient response: Metamorphose or die.

In the liminal space between comfort and crisis, the body remembers: Fasting depletes easy fuel - forces fat adaptation; Cold strips the artificial warmth – forces metabolic fire.

The vampire knows, discomfort is the whetstone of the soul. I have fasted in frozen rivers. Let hunger sharpen the cold's bite. Let cold deepen hunger's clarity. Modern man seeks one ritual. But the wild requires both. Skip a meal? Kill the heater. Hunt fasted? Hunt barefoot in snow.

Crossing both thresholds simultaneously? That's where alchemy lives. Fasted ice plunges shock the system into ketotic clarity. Your cells scream... then sing. It's not endurance. It's remembering. Thresholds are crossed alone. But on the other side, you meet the vampire you were before domestication.

Firewalker's Science

This isn't biohacking. It's bone memory:

- Fasting upregulates norepinephrine, cortisol and AMPK.
- Cold immersion at 14°C spiked norepinephrine 530% above baseline[1].
- Together, they synergize, boosting mitochondrial biogenesis via PGC-1α[7].
- Brown fat (BAT) ignites using UCP1, generating heat without shivering, a cellular bonfire[8].
- Cold-fasted bodies increase lipolysis by 287% compared to comfort-cloaked ones[2].

Cold-trained humans develop 300% more active BAT[5]. And cold shock proteins suppress inflammatory cytokines like IL-6 and TNF-α[6].

Wim Hof (The Iceman) trained subjects can suppress cytokine storms at will, proof that mitochondrial fire responds to command. You are the ritual and the result.

The Fire in the Ice - When Flesh Lights the Flame

Cold is not absence. It is ignition. Beneath your skin lies a sacred fuel: brown adipose tissue. In the cold, it lights. Uncoupling proteins (UCP1) disrupt the chain of ATP production, allowing energy to burn as heat. This is fire without flame, the same primal spark that lit ancestral eyes when hands plunged into steaming carcasses on frozen tundra. A hearth beneath your flesh.

Early humans knew this. Fire wasn't just survival; it was ritual transformation. The blaze was fed by death. The spark demanded offering.

I've lit fires in frozen caves and beneath skin, both fed by the same sacrifice. When the mammoth fell, it was dressed beside fire. The liver eaten raw. The fat fed to children.

But before all that, there was always the plunge. There was always the fast. Because the flame must be earned. UCP1 doesn't just burn fat; it uncouples survival from glucose.

Winter Child

They called her Sølvi, sun-strength in winter. She walked barefoot not for pain, but for pact. Her soles mapped the land's bones. When boys faltered, she'd press a sliver of frozen liver to their tongues: "Eat the cold. Become it." That liver held over 10,000 IU of vitamin A per gram[11], an Arctic nutrient, a metabolic sword.

She taught them to hunt fasted, stomachs empty, senses sharpened by frost. She carried no weapons. But the cold obeyed her. She wasn't a girl. She was winter's midwife, birthing hunters from softness. Her frozen blade foreshadowed the bone knife yet to come.

Marengo

I remember Marengo. Three nights. No food. The river frozen. Men prayed for warmth; I prayed for clarity. The taste of boiled leather, like burnt earth and despair. When the horse ribs cracked, marrow froze on my lips. I licked ice for water, salt for sanity.

Troops chewed leather to survive, not for calories but sodium, to fuel the cold-stressed pump. The cold carved hunger into a weapon.

You have not known yourself until you have starved in snow.

Cold and Ketones - A Double-Edged Memory Blade

Why do I still remember? Because cold and fasting protect what matters:

- Cold elevates ketones directly via the FGF21-PGC1α axis[3].
- Ketones upregulate BDNF, fueling cognitive resilience[4].

- Cold and ketones together preserve myelin, reduce oxidative stress and stimulate hippocampal neurogenesis[4].

This is biological cryopreservation. This is how the vampire remembers. Together, cold and fasting sculpt the brain as they do the body... lean, sharp, enduring. This is why my mind endures while yours frays. Why my thoughts strike with precision while yours drift. Because my forge never cooled.

Hunger Is a Forge

Comfort feeds decay. Hunger is a forge. A soft body is velvet-wrapped stone, useless for cutting. You were not made for plush chairs and snack packs. You were made for killing in snow. Presence is the blood that remembers.

You will remember the crack of ice on empty skin. The silence inside the shudder. The iron taste of your own thawing blood. The electric silence when cells ignite their inner forge.

The vampire remembers the frostbite that birthed him, and the hunger that saved him. You will not be the same when you step out.

Fast until your cells ignite. Freeze until your fat becomes a hymn. Take the plunge. Let glacial marrow be your communion.

You are forged in frost and baptized in flame

Chapter 19

The Blood of the Child

Raising Firekeepers in a Sugar-Coated Cage.

You were not born a feeder. You were born a firekeeper.
To raise a child is not to fill a bowl. It is to pass on the
flame. And yet ... we feed them like prisoners. We raise
them like cattle. We call it care, but it is sedation.

The vampire does not raise sheep. He raises wolves. And
so must you.

The Soft Cage

There was a time when children were carved by nature.
Their muscles shaped by hills, their bones hardened by
sun, their minds sharpened by silence and hunger.

Now they are raised indoors. Wrapped in Wi-Fi, softened
by snacks, praised for obedience and punished for
instinct. We feed them sugar and say it is love. We
medicate their wildness and call it care. We dress them in
softness and mourn when they break.

But what breaks them is not the world. It is the lie. The lie
that says children must be safe, not strong. That they must
be kept full, not forged hungry. That they are porcelain,
not firewood. Porcelain breaks. Firewood burns.

By fifteen, 24% of US teenagers already show prediabetes[1], not from living, but from the lie. And so we forget. The predator does not coddle its young. It teaches them to track, to kill, to feast, and to wait.

The Blood Memory

There is something ancient in a child. Before the screens, before the sugar, before the spell, there is memory. A blood memory. Of marrow sucked from bones. Of liver shared beneath moonlight. Of the thrill of the hunt, even if only imagined. This memory is not taught. It is triggered. By taste. By touch. By fire.

You give a child real meat, and their eyes change. The body remembers. The jaw reawakens. The soul stirs. They don't know what to call it. But the vampire does. It is return.

Sugar Is Not Love

They told you love was cupcakes. That celebration meant frosting. That birthdays meant glucose. That a child's joy was measured in grams of carbohydrates. But this was not tradition. This was addiction.

Modern children consume 19 teaspoons of sugar daily[2], triple ancestral intake. Their dopamine receptors are drowning in frosting.

Historically, the child's feast was meat. The initiation was liver. The sacred food was fat.

Among the Maasai, boys drink blood before their rite of passage. Their hemoglobin averages 15.9 g/dL[3]. No anemia in blood-fed boys.

Among the Inuit, children are weaned onto seal blubber and raw fish[4].

Among the Hadza, the first shared kill is an event of reverence[5].

Among the Spartans, boys were underfed on purpose so they would learn to steal, to fight, and to value strength over fullness[6].

And Roman legend holds that Romulus and Remus, twin founders of empire, were nursed by a she-wolf. Suckled not in cribs, but in caves[7].

They did not get gold stars for oat milk. They got praise for strength, fire, and survival. And the vampire watched all of it. Not as myth, but memory.

Because sugar is not love. Sugar is a muzzle stitched with frosting. It quiets the child's fire. It smooths their wild edges. It replaces initiation with sedation. To love a child is not to sweeten them. It is to sharpen them.

The Kid Who Killed

They called him too quiet. Too strange. He watched animals, not cartoons. He played with bones, not plastic. And he asked questions the adults couldn't answer.

One day, he came home with blood on his hands. A rabbit. Killed with a rock. Skinned with a stick.

They screamed. Scolded. Sent him to therapy. But his grandfather, old and nearly forgotten, took him aside. "What did you feel?" The boy looked up. "Hungry. Alive." The old man nodded. "Then don't let them take that from you."

The boy grew. Never killed for sport. But never feared the wild again. He became a doctor. Then a father. And when his daughter turned ten, he gave her a knife. Not to harm. But to remember. The kill is not violence. It is sacred reciprocity.

The child who learns to kill does not become a monster. He becomes hunter and healer.

Feeding the Flame

Liver is not punishment. It is a gift. Salt is not bad. It is necessary. Sunlight is not a threat. It is command. If you want your child to thrive, stop feeding them fear. Feed them what their bones crave:

- Fat for hormones
- Meat for growth
- Salt for Neurons
- Sun for mitochondria
- Fire for spirit
- Hunger for patience (fasting until true appetite)
- Cold for resilience

Liver provides retinol for eyesight, not beta-carotene guesswork[8]. Children convert less than 5% of plant-based beta-carotene to active vitamin A, but absorb 90%+ from liver[9].

This is not 'clean eating.' This is ancestral fueling. And the vampire knows, because he has raised tribes. Children who are fed like beasts do not become beasts. They become leaders.

And if you need proof, watch what happens when a child chews liver by firelight. The heat rising from the cast iron. The tang of blood and salt. The way they slowly chew, look up, eyes wide. Not with guilt, but with recognition. They are not just eating. They are remembering.

The Domestication Spell

Schools serve industrialized betrayal in plastic trays: seed oils to inflame, grains to enslave, sugar to sedate. 68% of school meal fats come from linoleic acid-rich oils[10]. Omega-6 bombs for developing brains. They call it 'balanced.' But it is not balance. It is sedation. Recess replaced the forest. Grains replaced guts. Obedience replaced instinct.

By twelve, their teeth are dull. By fourteen, their fire is gone. By eighteen, they bleat. And still, we ask: Why are they anxious? Why do they crave chaos? Why do they cut themselves?

Because we never taught them to cut meat. Because we never fed them the truth. This is not parent-shaming. It is system-burning.

The cage was built by corporations, not caregivers.

The Rewilded Child

You want your child to glow? Don't give them affirmations. Give them animal fat. Don't protect them from hard things. Expose them, gradually, fiercely, lovingly. Let them:

- Fast until they feel it
- Eat until they roar
- Sweat in sun
- Sleep in dark
- Climb trees tall enough to scare them
- Speak with fire

A child who fasts until noon and plays barefoot in frost activates brown fat three times faster than adults[11]. They don't need more rules. They need more rites. They don't need therapy. They need thresholds.

A child who grows without a kill will look for one elsewhere. Give them a ritual, or they'll create a rebellion.

The Son of Ashes

He was born in winter. Raised on bone broth and blood. Never knew a microwave. Only fire. The elders whispered, "Too much sun. Too much meat. He'll grow wild." He did.

At ten, he tracked deer. At twelve, he fasted under stars. At fifteen, his words were flint on stone. When he left, he left a knife on the hearth. Not as threat. But as promise. To return. To protect. To pass on the flame.

The child you raise with fire will one day become the fire.

Vampires Don't Feed Babies Cereal

I have seen empires fall for lack of iron. I have seen lineages rot from seed oil and syrup. I have seen the fire go out behind children's eyes. But I have also seen it return. In liver-fed infants. In fat-fed daughters. In sons who eat steak and climb trees and question everything.

You say, "kids are hard to feed." I say you forgot how to lead. They don't want nuggets. They want truth. And your job is not to fill their plate. It is to light their torch.

I showed Genghis Khan how marrow ignites empires. His warriors conquered on Biltong and blood.

The knife you give your daughter is Sølvi's frozen blade, thawed in ancestral fire. The knife is not a weapon. It is the firekeeper's tool.

The Lunchbox and the Lie

You were not weaned on wheat. The child's first food, before the blender, before the bib, was flesh. Liver mashed with mother's milk. Fat from marrow. Broth from bone. Across continents and centuries, infants were not softened. They were initiated.

Inuit weanlings consumed 10,000 IU of vitamin D per day from seal fat[12]. Modern lunchboxes average 98 IU from fortified snacks.

Among the Mongols, toddlers gnawed on dried mutton fat. Sun-dried, wind-cured, life-giving[4]. There were no snack packs. No organic pouches. No smiley-face carrots. Just blood, fat, fire, and the bones of beasts.

Now we hand them a lunchbox filled with betrayal. Plastic-wrapped granola, fortified crackers, lab-made yoghurts, soy-laced "meat-free" bites. A banana. Maybe a note. "Have a great day, sweetie!" But there is no greatness in that box. Only glucose. Only obedience.

A lunchbox is not love. A school meal is not sacred. A snack is not a rite. And until we reclaim the kill, we raise them as prey.

Hooves and Horses

There is a wind that does not forget. It howls across the steppes of Mongolia, past yurts stitched from felt and bone, through herds of shaggy horses and the fires of nomad camps. Here, children are not raised. They rise.

Among the Dukha reindeer herders, children ride at eighteen months[13]. By three, they drink fermented mare milk. By five, they help butcher goats with knives they are expected to respect but never fear.

Rural Mongolian children show one-third less asthma than their urban peers[14]. They also have 300% higher vitamin D than city kids[15]. They graze on strength. To grow up Mongolian is to grow up in motion. To be shaped by hooves, wind, and meat.

It is not romantic. It is real. No soft toys. No gluten-free guilt. Just the bone, the blood, the knife, and the sky.

The Daughter Who Lit the Knife

She was small. Too wild for their cage, they said. Too gentle. Too dreamy. Too much like her mother, before her mother forgot how to burn.

They gave her flax crackers and oat milk. They told her not to run too fast. They said she was sensitive. And she was. But not to feelings. To lies.

One day, she found her grandfather's knife. She carried it to the woods. She did not stab. She did not cut. She dug. She boiled water. She caught nothing but bugs, but she watched how they moved.

She returned, not with blood, but with questions. "What did we used to eat?" "Why did Nana stop hunting?" "Why do I feel stronger in the sun?" No one answered. But she knew.

The next week, she asked for steak. The next month, she carried firewood without complaint.

And the next year, when a boy said girls should be skinny, she looked him in the eye and said, "Only prey need to shrink."

And in her eyes, her mother saw her own mother again. Before the forgetting. Before the sugar.

A girl given fat will not fall for flattery. A girl given fire will not fear the dark.

Closing Invocation

And now I say to you. Put down the juice box. Pick up the knife. Feed your child the blood they crave. Not the sugar they're sold. And you will not raise a problem. You will raise a predator. You will not raise obedience. You will raise remembrance. Because you were never meant to raise a sheep. You were meant to raise the future. In blood. In bone. In flame. Let the fire return. Let the child remember. Let the blood of the child be not sugar. But strength. For the child is not a feeder to be filled. The child is the firekeeper, born to carry the flame.

Chapter 20

The Fire That Doesn't Bleed

*She is not aftermath; she is the ember that outlives the wildfire.
Her fire is no longer pulled by tides or time but burns inward.*

The Turning

The bleeding stops. The world doesn't. If anything, it sharpens.

They called her past it. Spent. Dried up. But they were wrong. She is not aftermath; she is the ember that outlives the wildfire. She no longer bleeds with the moon. She burns like the sun. Steady. Merciless. Sustaining.

For centuries, this transition has been framed as collapse. A falling off the cliff of youth. An exile from fertility. The end of the story.

But what if it's the beginning?

The Myth of the Dried Crone

Culture has made a ritual of shaming the menopausal woman. She is hidden, mocked, silenced. Her hormones drop. So does her social value. Her skin dries. So does the desire around her. Her womb closes. So do the doors of opportunity. And yet, in myth, she is more powerful than ever.

She becomes Hecate, walking between worlds. Kali, wielding destruction and rebirth. Baba Yaga, feral and wise in her forest of bones. And Yelena, the Bone-Faced One, whose face was not decay, but tusk carved by truth. Her voice cracked glaciers into rivers. Her rage bent seasons.

These are not broken women. They are the unbreakable spine of the feminine arc.

Hormones of Fire

Menopause is not hormone loss. It's metabolic rewiring. Estradiol doesn't simply disappear; it drops to liberate. Progesterone declines to shift the fire inward. What once flowed in service of fertility now flows in service of sovereignty.

The ovaries quiet, and the liver becomes the hormone factory. Cholesterol transforms into pregnenolone, then into adrenal DHEA: fueling clarity instead of fertility[6].

Mitochondria cease scattering energy for reproduction. They consolidate, holding fire for wisdom[1]. This is not entropy. It is mitophagy... the elegant burning of the broken, so that only the strong remain[7].

The system no longer stores fat for potential offspring. It begins to burn. To clarify. To refine.

Ketones rise. Fog lifts. The brain stops chasing and starts watching. Memory deepens. Mood stabilizes. A different kind of hunger emerges, one no longer tied to the tides of estrogen, but to something far older and something far more patient.

Feeding the Brain, Bone, and Flame

These hormonal shifts are not a curse. They are signals, asking you to fuel differently. To eat not for reproduction, but for cognition. Not for sweetness, but for signal.

Carnivore is not a diet; it is a remembering. One that feeds the post-fertile body with exactly what it needs:

- Saturated fat for hormone production
- Cholesterol, the raw material of sex hormones[2]
- Salt to regulate the adrenals during transition[8]
- Collagen to preserve joints and elasticity
- Protein to retain lean mass and bone density[3]

Data now affirms what instinct already knew: Postmenopausal women on carnivore diets show a 22.3% increase in insulin sensitivity and a marked reduction in inflammation[4]. Bone loss slows. Energy returns. Hot flashes subside.

Carnivore diets reduce menopausal hot flashes by 71% in clinical observation[5]... a metabolic calm, not suppression.

A 2021 study[9] found women eating a high-fat, animal-based diet had significantly stronger bones than peers on plant-based protocols. These aren't outliers. They are ancestors reclaiming flame.

Warning: Those with iron overload disorders (e.g., hemochromatosis) should limit organ consumption[10].

The Vampire Watches

I have lived a thousand years, but I do not understand this fire. I've seen kings fall, temples crumble, blood running in rivers, but nothing like her.

She loses her cycle and gains a stillness I cannot touch. I feast on youth. She holds its ghost in her marrow. I drink blood. She is the source.

Her fire mirrors my hunger, but hers is self-contained ignition. She needs no external fuel. Her marrow is her elixir. They say she is post-reproductive. I say she is post-illusion.

Her fire does not flicker. It incinerates illusion. Her mitochondria don't chase; they consolidate. While my hunger is eternal, hers is enough.

The Crone Ascends

You were not meant to fade. You were meant to flare.

They called it 'the change', as if it were a side street off the main road of womanhood. But it is not a deviation. It is the summit. This isn't the soft landing of decline. It's the summit of sovereignty.

Her skin thickens, not to protect, but to remember. Her sleep deepens, not from fatigue, but from calibration. Her appetite shifts, not from deficiency, but from discipline.

She no longer lives by the clock. She lives by the kill. She drinks marrow, the unapologetic sap of sovereignty. She eats liver. She salts her flesh. She walks barefoot. She does not fear menopause. She 'meats' it. She answers with flesh. She has reclaimed her cells' ancestral memory; the patience of predators who know stillness fuels the pounce.

The Woman Who Waited

They called her barren. She smiled.

Every month, for forty years, she had bled. She had fed husbands, children, and jobs. But now her blood was her own. The tide had turned inward. No longer did it flow down and out. It circled. And in the silence that followed, something moved.

At first it felt like loss. Then it felt like space. Then it felt like fire. Her fasts weren't starvation; they were mitochondrial recalibration. Her feast: bison heart, sea salt, sunlight.

Her hair silvered, her skin thickened, her voice dropped. She stopped apologizing for any of it.

They called her barren. But it was her emptiness that held the sun.

The Fire Doesn't Fade

They will try to tame it. They will sell hormone patches. Antidepressants. Plastic smiles and soy-based serenity. But this is not a deficiency. It is a divergence.

The modern world cannot comprehend the Crone. She does not entertain. She does not smile for tips. She does not fit in your demographic funnel.

She sharpens knives and forgets birthdays. She tells the truth and burns bridges. And she eats like a predator. No sugar. No apologies. No famine foods. She is fat-fueled, flame-bound, and frost-hardened.

She remembers what famine taught and refuses to repeat it. She does not gather. She hunts. She does not whimper. She waits. She does not fear menopause. She 'meats' it.

The Midwife Who Burned

She had delivered 417 babies. Then she was exiled for the one she didn't.

The mother bled too fast. The child had crowned too slowly. The priest called it punishment. The mayor called it witchcraft. She called it time.

In exile, she found the mountain cave. It was dry and high, and nobody visited. That suited her. There, she bled her last. There, her fire began.

She ate nothing but bone broth and salted meat. She watched the stars. She slept with a knife. Her mountain cave was a frost-forged sanctuary. Cold sharpened her fast. Marrow deepened her sight.

Over time, they came to her. The young, the sick, the childless. They brought liver and questions. She gave back marrow and answers. They called her cursed. But something in her silence became flame.

The Law of the Crone

The young bleed with the moon. The Crone burns with the sun. She no longer cycles. She sears. She does not flow. She holds. She does not chatter. She carves.

Her mitochondria stopped chasing. They hold. Her rituals are fewer. Her memory is longer. She does not wait for permission. She makes fire from hunger. She fasts like a glacier, slow, inevitable, carving truth from stone. She feasts like a wildfire, devouring darkness, leaving only light. She walks barefoot. She speaks rarely. She remembers everything.

The young bleed with the moon. The wise burn with the sun. You are not fading. You are forging. Never apologize for the fire that doesn't bleed.

Chapter 21

The Misfit's Hunger

They diagnosed your memory as madness. But your hunger was not broken. It was ancestral.

The Vampire Was Never Normal

He never liked crowds. He blinked too slowly. Stared too long. Heard things others didn't. He avoided the banquet. Hid from the sun. Slept when the world woke. And when he spoke, it wasn't casual. It was sacred. Rare. Ritual.

To the herd, he seemed strange. Antisocial. Difficult. A sacred misfit. But he wasn't broken. He remembered hunger before snacks, fire before comfort, instinct before etiquette. He remembered a time when the senses were not dulled by screens and sedatives, but sharpened by silence, fasting, and the hunt.

The vampire was not a villain. He was a neurodivergent ancestor with metabolic clarity. A being who had refused the sedation of the simulation. So are you.

The Stimmers, the Dreamers, and the Ones Who Never Fit

They called you too much. Too loud. Too quiet. Too fast. Too slow. Too intense. Too distracted. They tested your attention span. Scored your speech patterns. Monitored your fidgeting. Graphed your eye contact.

Then they gave it a name: ADHD. Autism. Bipolar. OCD. Tourette's. Sensory Processing Disorder. A pathology for every part of you that didn't fit their factory. But what if it wasn't pathology?

What if your so-called disorder was a preserved ancestral function, one that civilization has no use for, but evolution refused to delete?

Your stimming is ritual, unbroken lineage from fire-tenders and star-readers. Your hyperfocus is a hunting trance. Your silence is sacred restraint. Your resistance is ancestral instinct. Your brain isn't damaged. It's different because it's older.

The brain you have is not broken. It is a message in a bottle from a wilder time.

The Ancient Roles of the Neurodivergent Mind

In ancestral tribes, not everyone was a hunter with a spear. Some were pattern-seers. Star-trackers. Bone-readers.

The boy who fixated on how shadows moved across rock became the tribe's navigator. The girl who refused conversation but listened to wolves became a warning bell. The child who couldn't sit still but could track a deer for hours became the best stalker. The one who avoided touch and obsessed over fire became the shaman. The one who never slept at night? The night sentinel, the one who heard what others missed. The child who rocks? They're keeping time like a shaman's drum.

Autistic pattern-seers detected threats 0.3 seconds faster than neurotypicals[11]. ADHD hyperfocus enabled 36% longer endurance during visual tracking tasks[12]. The vampire's 'rigid rituals? Sacred precision. His 'avoidant' traits? Night-sentinel vigilance.

Today, these same traits are called disorders. But the vampire remembers when they were sacred. He doesn't fit into classrooms. He doesn't follow meal schedules. He waits, watches, fasts, and remembers.

The Rise of the Diagnostic Cage

The DSM, Diagnostic and Statistical Manual of Mental Disorders, is not a book of truth. It is a colonial taxonomy for wild brains. A catalogue of inconvenient instincts. It lists symptoms like:

- Difficulty with transitions
- Resistance to authority
- Repetitive interests
- Unusual sensory response
- Preference for solitude
- Obsession with movement
- Fixation on ritual

But what if these aren't flaws? What if these are preserved instincts? What if these are the traits that once kept your tribe alive?

DSM 'symptoms' were once survival traits. Resistance to authority prevented poisoned grain consumption. Sensory overwhelm detected forest fires miles away. The DSM doesn't name your pain. It names your refusal to comply. It pathologizes your hunger for silence, movement, meaning. And then... it medicates it.

The DSM pathologizes the hunter in a farmer's world.

Medicated Minds, Malnourished Souls

You walk into a clinic. You say:

> "I feel restless."
> "I can't focus."
> "I hate small talk."
> "I can't eat this food."
> "I can't sleep under lights."
> "I feel everything too much."
> "I feel nothing at all."

And the answer is always the same: "Here. Take this". SSRIs. Benzos. Antipsychotics. Amphetamines. Chemical leashes for wild minds. The doctor doesn't ask: What do you eat? Do you fast? Do you sit in silence? Do you crave ritual? Does the modern world feel hostile because it is? He hands you a script, a map to nowhere.

But the vampire doesn't take scripts. He fasts. He feeds. He listens to his hunger. You cannot medicate away a sacred mind's cry for remembrance.

This isn't anti-medication. It's pro-metabolic choice. Some need pharmaceuticals. But all deserve ancestral nourishment.

The Carnivore Brain: Reclaiming Neurochemical Sovereignty

The neurodivergent brain is metabolically unique. Energy-hungry. Mitochondrially fragile. Often inflamed by modern food.

- Cholesterol scaffolds the myelin sheath that insulates and accelerates neural signals. Low cholesterol slows conduction by up to 50% in ADHD[13].
- Saturated animal fat supports dopamine synthesis and stabilizes reward circuits[14].
- Linoleic acid, the seed oil molecule found in "heart-healthy" foods, oxidizes in the amygdala, increasing anxiety by up to 300%[15].
- Ketones bypass glucose metabolism, soothing overstimulated neural pathways, reducing glutamate toxicity, and enhancing clarity[2].
- 68% of autistic brains show mitochondrial fragmentation, reversible through ketogenic interventions[16].
- Glycine, abundant in bone broth, balances GABA-glutamate ratios, easing sensory overwhelm[17].

This isn't fringe. This is metabolic psychiatry[8]. For many, the answer isn't Prozac. It's steak, salt, and silence.

Neurodivergence is not a glitch. It's a message. It says: "The simulation is unlivable. Return to ritual."

The Firechild

She never spoke in class. Never raised her hand. Bit her knuckles. Screamed at bells. Flapped her hands when no one was looking.

They gave her pills. She stopped screaming. But she stopped humming too.

Then one day, a strange man arrived. He carried no clipboard. Only a pouch of dried liver and a flask of bone broth. He sat beside her. He said nothing. She crawled to him like a wolf cub to alpha, instinct recognizing instinct. He gave her meat. She chewed. She smiled.

And for the first time in years… she hummed. A low, deep, perfect tone. The room fell still.

He handed her another bite. And the humming never stopped. She wasn't stimming. She was drumming. Her hum was the ancestral echo of the kill.

The Hungry Brain Is Not a Broken Brain

Let's be clear: Neurodivergent people are not broken neurotypicals. They are different. Older. Sharper in some places, softer in others. They crave honesty; rhythm; stillness; meaning; pattern and… meat!

Their nervous systems are porous. Their metabolism craves ancestral coal. They can't lie. They can't fake. They can't tolerate processed noise. This isn't disorder. This is signal.

Hunger Is Not a Symptom. It's a Compass.

You crave movement. You crave ritual. You crave fat, salt, silence. These aren't compulsions. They are remembrance. The stim is the smoke from a fire not yet lit. Your craving is the compass. The resistance is the roar.

For those who carry this ancestral memory, hunger is your compass. But the world says suppress. So, you chew plastic. Tap screens. Swallow pills. And the fire dims. Until one day… you remember.

The Night of the Fire Feast

He hated parties. Loathed eye contact. Fled meetings like prey. Took his meds. Ate his lentils. Still felt wrong.

Then one night, a message arrived: "The fire still walks. Come hungry." He did.

In the hills, around a bone-lit table, they ate. Meat. Liver. Marrow. Salt. No words. No screens. No judgment. Only fire. Only flesh. Only memory. And he wept, salt and fire merging on his lips, because he was home.

Ritual for the Remembering Mind

You don't need fixing. You need the hunt. You need:

- Fasting - for silence
- Feasting - for strength
- Fire - for memory
- Salt - for clarity
- Meat - for fuel
- Movement - not gyms, but exile from the screen
- Stillness - not laziness, but listening
- Fire-gazing - for trance states that rewire default mode networks

The Misfit's Plate

Eat like the firekeeper you are:

- Liver daily - Retinol for light-sensitive eyes
- Bone broth fasting - Glycine calms glutamate storms
- Zero seed oils - Starve the linoleic acid inflammation
- Salt to taste - Sodium for electrical clarity
- Avoid high-oxalate plants - Oxalates whisper like glass inside overstimulated synapses[18]

The carnivore diet isn't a trend for you. It's metabolic repatriation.

Vampiric Monologue

I have seen what they call you. Disorder. Spectrum. Delay. Deficit. But I know who you are.

You are the one who flinches at lies. Who stims because stillness kills you. Who rages against the noise because your cells remember the silence. Who bites your arm because the world is too fake, too loud, too slow.

I know you. Because I am you. Not broken. Just remembered. You are flame-fed, bone-carved, and meat-bound. You are the unbitten fruit of an ancient tree.

You Are Not Alone

You were told to sit still. To speak softly. To medicate your hunger. To apologize for your edge.

But I say: You are not a problem. You are a memory. You are not unwell. You are uncolonized. You are not too much. You are too rare. You are not a diagnosis. You are a signal. Your 'meltdowns' are metabolic revolt. Your 'obsessions' are ancestral focus. Your brain isn't disordered. It's disproportionately alive.

Not every neurodivergent person will resonate with the hunter metaphor. That is the beauty of neural biodiversity. You are one of us. You are the Misfit. The Firechild. The Flame That Remembers. Now tend the flame.

Chapter 22

The Vampire's Code

Discipline is sovereignty. Build your rituals. Fast like a mystic.
Feast like a god. Sleep like a wolf. The vampire thrives because he
obeys the laws of instinct, not culture.

The Hunger for Order

We romanticize freedom. But the vampire knows the
truth… freedom without form is chaos. A predator
without discipline is a liability, to himself, to his clan, to
the hunt. The vampire does not wake by whim or eat by
clock. He obeys rhythm, not regulation. He follows code,
not commandment. And it is this obedience, not to
culture, but to instinct, that grants him his power.

The modern human, by contrast, has confused liberation
with license. Eat when you want. Sleep when you're tired.
Train when you're motivated. This is not freedom. This is
entropy perfumed as self-actualization.

Discipline is not denial. It is devotion to a future self. The
vampire does not live impulsively. He lives in ceremony.
And so must you.

The Loss of the Code

Modern culture treats discipline as pathology. It
pathologizes discipline because a structured mind is

ungovernable. The dopamine economy relies on your disorder. Fasting is subversive. Stillness is a threat. Your morning walk? Drowned in autoplay. Your ritual? Hijacked by an algorithm addicted to your fragmentation.

The school teaches compliance, not rhythm. The gym teaches reps, not ritual. The doctor prescribes pills, not process. And the result? Disordered lives. Disordered eating. Disordered sleep. Lives without gravity.

Discipline is not control. It is context. It is the architecture that allows your instinct to thrive. It is the way the predator remembers who he is in a world that keeps asking him to forget.

The Herd's Lie: "Routines are rigid." The Vampire's Truth: "Rituals are metabolic rivers; they carve canyons through the sedimentary lies of snack culture."

The Boy Without the Code

He was praised for being 'free.' No rules. No bedtime. No boundaries. He ate when hungry, played when bored, slept when tired. He was the experiment of an enlightened age: unshaped, unshackled, undone.

But the freedom turned sour. Without rhythm, he grew restless. Without rules, he grew wild, but not strong. He snacked constantly. Fidgeted through nights. Feared the dark but hated the light.

One day, the world broke. The digital scaffold fell. And the boy, now grown, now hollow, was cast out. Alone in the wild, he was found by a man cloaked in night. A vampire. But not the monster he'd imagined. The vampire fed him not blood, but bone broth. Salt. Silence.

He made him wait. He taught him to fast. To breathe cold air at dawn. To eat in firelight. To move before eating. To sleep in rhythm with the dark. The boy resisted. Then yielded. Then remembered.

And years later, when asked what saved him, he said: "Not the vampire's rules. But that he had them." Discipline is not oppression. It is the framework of freedom. Without a code, even the wildest heart becomes prey.

The Metabolic Mandate: Why Discipline Heals

Modern science now confirms what vampires and monks already knew: structure heals. Circadian biology, the 24-hour clock embedded in your genes, governs everything from hormone release to insulin sensitivity. And it demands discipline.

Eating late disrupts leptin and melatonin, impairing sleep and fat metabolism[1]. It increases leptin resistance by 58% and reduces fat oxidation by 27%[2]. Skipping morning light exposure delays cortisol, making you foggy and inflamed[3]. Dawn light boosts cortisol amplitude by 40%, reducing systemic inflammation[4]. Inconsistent bedtimes wreck

REM cycles and impair memory[5]. Going to sleep at 10 p.m. consistently increases free testosterone by 28%[6].

Time-restricted feeding (TRF), especially when aligned with daylight hours, improves glucose control, lowers inflammation, and restores mitochondrial biogenesis through PGC-1α[7]. In carnivore-specific studies, an 8-hour TRF reduced HbA1c by 0.8% and increased ketones to 2.1 mmol/L[8].

Unlike the mythic vampire, your cells are sun-bound creatures. You are not meant to feed in the dark. Fasting before exercise boosts fat oxidation and elevates growth hormone[9]. Fasted movement increases lipolysis threefold compared to fed training[10]. In neurodivergent populations, TRF has reduced ADHD symptoms by 40%[11].

Deep sleep is when testosterone rises, not by chemical accident, but by lunar design. It's the hour of repair. Autophagy clears debris[12] like a predator cleaning bone. The glymphatic system washes the brain's battlefield, rinsing neural waste from the day's hunt[13]. Deep sleep also clears amyloid-beta 60% faster than wakefulness[14].

Sleep isn't rest. It's ritual restoration. Structure is your supplement.

The Predator's Rhythm: Fast, Feast, Move, Sleep

The vampire lives by the fourfold code of metabolic sovereignty:

Fast like a mystic: Hunger is not an error. It is a signal. Fasting trains metabolic flexibility, sharpens cognition, and awakens ancient pathways of survival[15]. It increases norepinephrine by 200% and elevates BDNF by 50%[16].

Feast like a god: When you eat, eat without fear. Meat, fat, salt, no apology. Feasting post-fast increases nutrient absorption, resets appetite hormones, and strengthens reward circuitry. It also sustains dopamine in a way snacking never could[17].

Move before eating: Movement in a fasted state, especially walking, lifting, sprinting, triggers a primal cascade: BDNF, AMPK, growth hormone[18]. The predator earns his kill.

Sleep like a wolf: Cold, dark, and early. Block blue light, drop your body temp, rise with the sun. Sleep like Sølvi's winter wolves: still-bodied, senses blazing.

Discipline as Identity, Not Punishment

The modern mind views discipline as a burden. But to the vampire, and to the sovereign, it is identity.

You are not disciplined because you hate yourself. You are disciplined because you remember yourself.

The Maasai warrior doesn't graze. He drinks blood and walks for hours, because his body remembers the code of the savannah: Move or starve. Feast or fail.

The samurai's tea ceremony before battle isn't mere ritual. It's neural priming. The stillness isn't aesthetic. It's cortisol control, glucose alignment, pre-kill precision. Samurai tea ceremony has been shown to reduce cortisol by 32%[19]. By contrast, modern "mindfulness apps" increase cognitive load by 41%[20].

These aren't habits. They're ancestral physiology in prayer. Discipline is a declaration. It says: "I choose structure because I am not prey." It says: "I fast because my ancestors did." It says: "I do not chase energy. I channel it." This isn't perfectionism, it's pulse-finding. Miss a ritual? Return like the tide: relentless, unhurried, ancestral.

Your rhythm is unique. Arctic nightwalkers need different code than desert sun-hunters. Listen to your mitochondria. You were not born for freedom alone. You were born for rhythm.

I Am the Code

I do not wake by accident. I rise in darkness. I drink water, salt, and silence. I do not snack. I wait. I do not train when convenient. I train when required. I do not need motivation. My mitochondria have memory. I remember what the herd forgot. That freedom without form is starvation. That power without pattern is wasted.

I fast because I am fire. I feast because I have earned it. I move because the body demands obedience. I sleep because the kill is complete. I breathe because the night demands it. I breathe because nasal nitric oxide increases 600% in dawn air, sterilizing lungs, fueling mitochondria[21]. I do not bend to comfort. I do not obey convenience. I do not chase novelty. I keep the code.

Because I remember the hunger that made me. And I will not trade that hunger for softness. Not now. Not ever.

The Discipline of the Undying

Discipline is not rigidity. It is remembrance. Of fire. Of rhythm. Of the way your blood once moved before algorithms sedated it. Your 'distraction' is sensory vigilance, hijacked by apps that crave your fragmentation.

The vampire does not crave rules. He keeps them. Because in a world that is crumbling, code is the only thing that endures. Build your rituals:

- Wake with the sun.
- Walk before eating.
- Fast in the quiet.
- Feast in the fire.
- Sleep like a wolf, all muscle and moon, no apology.

Let them mock your stillness. Let them fear your consistency. Let them crumble beneath chaos.

You? You walk the code. Because you remember. Because you are not broken. You are structured. Because you are not impulsive. You are instinctual. You are not a slave to feelings. You are a creature of fire and law. You are the vampire, the unbitten, the unfragmented, the unapologetic keeper of the flame that modernity tried to extinguish.

And the code is your flame.

Chapter 23

Organs and Ancestors

The sacred kill bleeds across centuries. Your teeth are the fate-line connecting Halvar's first heart to your last. The flesh is not food. It is fire passed down. To eat the heart is to remember the hands that once hunted.

The Blood Rite Begins

The boy had eaten no flesh for three days. No words passed his lips. Only bone broth. Only salt. Only silence.

At sunrise, they painted his chest with brine and soot. At dusk, with blood. Not to anoint him, but to remember him. To mark who he was before the kill.

Halvar knelt by the fire, not as a hunter, but as a vessel. Around him, the men of the steppe stood cloaked in smoke and scar tissue. Their eyes did not shine. They burned.

The elder placed the heart of a stag before him, still raw, still warm. He spoke not in command, but covenant: "This is not meat. It is memory. It is the beat your ancestors followed through winter. The drum they fed on when the sun would not rise. The muscle that never lied."

Halvar bowed. He did not chew with hunger. He chewed with reverence. And in that moment, he ceased to be only himself. He became the sum of every hunter who came before him, and every hunger that had howled across the steppe.

Organs Are Not Cuts. They Are Covenant.

Modern people divide the body into cuts. Tenderloin. Ribeye. Sirloin. Chops.

But to the ancestral mind, these were not commodities. They were consequence. And the organs, heart, liver, brain, marrow, testicle - were never optional. They were sacred. The muscle fed the clan. The organs fed the fire.

In every carnivorous tribe, these sacred parts were consumed first and often by the eldest, the hunters, or the initiate. Not for vanity. For vitality. Because the organs were more than dense with nutrients. They were dense with meaning. To eat a liver is to signal the gods. To chew heart is to carry covenant. To suck marrow is to inherit the line. To eat testicle is to wake the flame.

These were not metaphors. They were biological truths wrapped in ancestral rites. Organs are metabolic heirlooms. Liver isn't food, it is liquid ancestry. Marrow isn't fat, it is cryogenized memory.

The Biochemistry of Memory

Let us now name the sacred pieces. And let the old proverbs lead the way.

Liver: The Keeper of the Flame

Liver holds retinol (true vitamin A), B12, copper, folate, choline, at densities unmatched by any plant, powder, or pill[1]. Just 100g of beef liver offers over 5,000% of your daily B12, and more bioavailable vitamin A than ten pounds of carrots[2].

It nourishes vision, fertility, detoxification, mitochondrial repair, and blood formation. It is not a "superfood." It is a biological telegram from your ancestry. A single bite can restore what a season of greens cannot. To ancestral peoples, liver was the first organ touched after the kill and often eaten raw, before the rest was even carved.

Taste the metallic tang on your tongue, the flavor of your own blood remembering itself. It was not dessert. It was divine inheritance.

Heart: The Drum That Fed the Fire

Heart offers CoQ10, taurine, selenium, and heme iron[3]. But more than that, it offers memory, rhythm, spirit. In many tribes, the heart was split among hunters or passed to the eldest son in raw slices. Not for protein. For remembrance. To eat the heart is to join its rhythm. To eat the heart is to become worthy of it.

Brain: The Eye Behind the Eyes

Brains are rich in DHA, phosphatidylserine, sphingomyelin, and cholesterol[4] - key to cognition, myelin repair, and hormonal balance.

Inuit and Mongol traditions treated brain not as hazard, but as hidden key - consumed with silence, reserved for the wise. Modern fear has masked it. But ancestral clarity demands it. To eat brain is to light the dark from within.

Note: In regions with BSE risk, avoid ruminant brains. Use ancestral alternatives such as bone marrow or fisheyes[5].

Marrow: The Song in the Bone

Marrow carries stem cell precursors, vitamin K2, conjugated linoleic acid, and deep ancestral fat[6]. Predators know this. They gnaw bones first. The hyena doesn't seek steak. She seeks memory.

Marrow is what endures when the flesh is gone. Marrow is the last hymn when the snow comes. Salt remembers the wound. Marrow remembers the winter.

Testicle: The Fire's Root

Testes contain pregnenolone (3.2 mg/g), cholesterol, vitamin A, and androgenic precursors[7]. They reignite vitality, rebuild hormone integrity, and rekindle the flame in the sedated. This is not performance enhancement. This is biological remembrance. To eat testicle is to defy softness

Biochemical Prayer - A Ritual for the First Bite

Before eating liver: "May this fire light my cells." Before heart: "May this drum beat in my blood." Before brain: "May these eyes guide my hunt."

These are not incantations. They are neurogastronomic triggers, priming digestion through reverence and awakening ancestral memory[8]. Reverent eating activates opioid receptors and increases mineral absorption by up to 70%[9]. Your prayer is not poetry. It is digestive enzymology.

Carnivorous Amnesia

Organ meats are now hidden. Covered in euphemism. Masked with shame. Relegated to capsules and sterilized pouches.

Why? Because modernity hides what forces us to confront death and our own animality. A steak in plastic wrap lets you forget the thud of the falling body. Liver on a Styrofoam tray lets you ignore the hands that carved it. This isn't convenience. It's carnivorous amnesia. And worse, desecration disguised as dinner.

The CAFO cow's liver isn't sacred. It's saturated with endotoxins and contains over 400% more PFAS than pasture-raised equivalents[10]. Its heart pumped antibiotics. Its marrow carries the ache of concrete and confinement.

CAFO livers also accumulate aflatoxins from GMO corn, causing triple the mitochondrial damage seen in wild game[11]. That's not food. That's a funeral for meaning.

The predator knows better. He does not abstract the sacred. He eats it.

Halvar Returns - The Sacred Kill

Three days later, Halvar stood at the edge of the gorge. The ibex below hadn't seen him. His bow was drawn. His breath, still. His limbs, steady. Not with bravado, but with remembrance.

He had fasted. He had trained. He had swallowed the symbols of strength. And now, it was time. The arrow flew. The kill was clean. The blood hissed on the snow, a final breath meeting winter.

The men came, not with applause, but with firelight and silence. They skinned the body with knives that were passed down, not purchased.

The liver was cut into five pieces: one for the elder; one for the earth; one for the ancestors; one burned as offering and one for the boy.

As Halvar took the final slice, a vision struck him. He saw eyes that were not his. He felt snow that was not this day. He heard wolves. He smelled smoke from another century. And then, he chewed. No fear. Only fire.

The elder placed a blooded hand on his shoulder. "You are no longer Halvar," he said. "You are Rauthr now, the Red One. Because you remembered."

Halvar's vision wasn't mysticism. It was ancestral DNA stirring. Exosomes from organ meats may awaken dormant pathways, igniting memory at the cellular level[12].

Do Not Waste the Sacred

I do not waste what bled for me. I do not cut around the truth and call it clean. I chew the parts you fear - heart, liver, blood, marrow. Because I do not flinch at death. I owe it everything.

I eat heart because I still have one. I eat liver because it remembers more than I do. I eat brain because I refuse sedation. I eat marrow because winter still comes. I eat testicles because softness starves the sacred.

You fear these foods because they make you remember. You've been taught to seek pleasure, not power. To seek comfort, not covenant. You hide organs in capsules while I chew them raw. Your supplement is sacrifice without communion.

My feast is covenant. But I remember. I remember the cold. I remember the blood. I remember the body that fed me. And I will not dishonor it with waste.

The Fire Returns

The organs are not excess. They are essence. To eat them is to honor the kill. To eat them is to say: "I see you. I thank you. I carry you forward."

You were not born into this ritual. But you can return to it. You have eaten no flesh for three days. You have swallowed salt and silence. You have waited by the fire. Now you remember.

The First Sacred Bite

Source grass-fed organs (liver or heart first). Salt generously. Chew slowly, eyes closed. Swallow not with gratitude, but with the recognition: This fire is ancestral. Now it is mine.

Eat like something sacred died for you …because it did.

Chapter 24

The Heart That Hides

Metabolic Exiles: How Carnivores Became 'Vampires' in a Grain-Worshipping World

We did not choose the shadows. We were banished to them. They said we drank blood. That we slept in coffins. That we couldn't enter a house unless invited. But what they didn't say, what they couldn't say, was that we were here first. That long before the age of plough and prayer, before domestication drained the fire from men's bones, we hunted the open lands, fed once a day, and walked in silence. We were not monsters. We were metabolic memory.

The vampire was born the day the last true carnivore was cast out, not with chains, but with stories. Turned into nightmare. Made taboo. Because when the fields rose, and the temples bloomed, and the grain grew tall, the flesh-eaters became inconvenient. We were too strong. Too quiet. Too fast to decay. And worst of all, we did not kneel.

The word vampire did not come from the West. Like the figure it names, it came from the cold earth of the East. Its roots are Slavic - *upir, wampir, opiri* - a tangled forest of tongues, from Bulgaria to Poland, Serbia to Hungary. It meant 'the one who drinks', 'the restless one', 'the thing that will not rot."

The earliest written record is from 1047, scrawled in Old Russian. But the myth is older than ink. It belonged to the folk, passed in whispers across the dark soil of the steppe[1].

In many versions, the vampire was not an evil aristocrat. It was a peasant who refused to die. A hunter found walking days after burial. A soldier who healed too quickly. A body dug up that smelled of nothing, with ruddy skin and blood at the lips. They burned those bodies. Not because they were afraid of evil, but because they were afraid of what the body remembered[1].

When the fields rose, the carnivores fell. The agricultural shift was not only a change in diet. It was a change in allegiance. To tame the land, one had to tame hunger. To build the temple, one had to forget the hunt. Agriculture wasn't cultivation. It was metabolic colonization. Ploughs cut steppes; sermons cut throats.

The meat-eaters, the real ones, were not needed in this new world. They didn't conform. They didn't ask permission. They lived on blood, fat, and silence.

So, the grain priests did what priests have always done. They turned hunters into horrors with three lies: Meat is murder. Fat is filth. Sovereignty is sin. The first genocide was metabolic. Hide your children. Burn the corpse. Fear the flesh.

But who really lived in darkness? The one who remembered the kill, or the one who learned to eat lightless bread under roofs they didn't build?

The Chinese chroniclers feared them. Not because they flew, but because they didn't stop. The Mongol warrior could ride for fourteen hours, eat once a day, live off horse blood, fermented milk, dried meat, and resolve[2]. They carried no grain, no baggage, no excuses. They healed fast. They slept little. They burned cities and vanished like smoke. One record notes: "They do not eat like men. They do not stop to rest. They are hard to kill. They are hunger made flesh." [2]

But they weren't spirits. They were carnivores. Modern forensic analysis confirms: ketotic preservation is real. Mongol graves show three times lower oxidative stress markers compared to contemporaneous agrarian populations[3]. Their bodies decayed more slowly. Ketones didn't just fuel their advance; they delayed their return to dust.

As their empire swept westward, through Slavic lands and into the trembling folds of Europe, their shadow left a scar. The people saw what they could not explain: lean men, scarless and silent, eating meat raw and walking through fire.

The myths wrote themselves. The OMAD discipline. The metabolic clarity. The ritual feasting. All lived in these horse-bound men. All feared by the grain-fed world. They said we drank blood. They weren't wrong. We drank it warm, from the throat of the hunt. Not because it was cursed, but because it was alive. Blood meant cholesterol, fat, iron - everything the brain craves, everything the temple fears.

What they never told you is that the vampire's blood is not a curse, it's a fuel. It is cholesterol. It is ketones. It is the liquid gold of the uninflamed mind[4]. It is not sugar that sustains us. It is sugar that swells, inflames, and rots. The vampire avoids glucose not out of superstition, but because he does not wish to decay.

Modern medicine would have you fear it. Fear fat. Fear red. Fear anything that does not come in a box.

But the vampire knows the truth. Cholesterol is memory. It is mood. It is the matrix of hormones and the cradle of clarity. Cholesterol is not a molecule. It's the molecule. The scaffold of sex, sanity, and sovereignty[5].

Even in medicine today, vampirism lives on. Not in folklore, but in metabolism. Glucose addiction is the new parasitism. And sugar is the only hunger that never sleeps.

They say we do not appear in mirrors. That's true. But not because we lack a soul. The mirror reflects the domesticated self, the jaw softened by bread, the eyes dimmed by fructose[6]. We stand behind the glass because we are the crack in it.

To see a vampire is to see yourself without the story. Without the grain. Without the lie. And that is what they feared most… that you might look into the darkness and see something real[7].

The Man Who Wouldn't Rot

They dug him up on the eleventh day. His name was Peter, or something close. He had died in the village of Kisilova, a small Balkan town clinging to the edge of night. No family claimed him. No priest buried him. He was just... gone.

But then the stories came. The farmer, whose daughter said she saw him in the field. The woman who swore she heard his boots outside her door. And then the cow that bled dry in the barn.

So, they exhumed him. And there he was. Skin red and full. Lips stained dark. Nails long, as if he had waited. A trickle of blood ran from the side of his mouth. The corpse was rosy and plump, with new skin under the nails. Described not with horror, but awe[8]. They staked him. Burned him. Buried what was left. But the question stayed. Why had he not rotted?

This was real. The year was 1725. The man was Peter Plogojowitz. The account was documented in an Austrian military report - still archived today. [8] Forensic re-evaluation suggests: His 'plumpness' could indicate anti-edema from low insulin. The 'new skin' may reflect extreme autophagy, cellular renewal through ketosis[9].

In Tibet, they tell a different story. Some monks, when they die, do not decay. Their bodies shrink, glow, or disappear entirely - leaving behind only hair and nails[10]. They are not feared. They are revered. Western science calls it autolysis resistance. The faithful call it rainbow body[11].

In 2002, the monk Khenpo Achö reportedly shrank to just 18 inches after death[10]. These reports remain anecdotal, but biochemically plausible. Whether grace or ketosis, incorruptibility challenges decay's inevitability.

Rainbow Body isn't magic. It's mitochondrial mastery. Tibetan monks exhibit elevated levels of chaperone mediated autophagy proteins (HSP70/BAG3), a cellular cleansing cascade triggered by deep fasting and a high-fat diet[12].

The monk and the vampire share the same metabolic pathway. Zero glucose, zero decay. And just like the vampire, these monks fasted in silence. Alone. In caves.

Both traditions share five non-negotiables:

1. OMAD feeding
2. Cold exposure (caves or steppes)
3. Zero plants
4. Circadian alignment
5. Ritual stillness

What if metabolic mastery, carnivorous solitude, and deep spiritual awareness do the same thing? What if the monk and the vampire are not opposites, but brothers?

What if both are proof that a human, given meat, fat, silence, and time, can become incorruptible? The vampire was not cast into darkness because he was evil. He was cast there because he did not kneel. He did not eat the grain. He did not wear the cloth. He did not rot when told.

So, they wrote him into the shadow. A myth. A monster. A whisper to scare children back to the table.

But we are still here. Still feeding on fat and memory. Still refusing to forget.

And you, dear reader, you have felt it. In the hunger behind your eyes. In the calm that returns when you eat only meat. In the dream that tastes like blood and truth. You feared the vampire because you feared yourself. One meal. No apologies. No inflammation. No lies.

We do not rise with the sun. We rise when the world forgets itself. We feed only when needed. We feel no shame. We walk without reflection because we carry no mask. We are not beasts. We are fossilized hunger sharpened into a blade.

You were told the vampire was a monster. That he lived in the dark. That he fed on the weak.

But what if he was simply the last man who remembered? What if the vampire was the carnivore who never converted? What if the darkness wasn't where he hid, but where he was banished?

And what if the only thing that can truly pierce him is the one thing no one dares offer anymore... a heart unafraid of its own hunger.

Chapter 25

The Infected Herd - Why the Vampire Didn't Cough

The Metabolic Fortress: Why Carnivores Walk Unscathed Through Pandemics

The streets were silent, but the shelves were not. Pasta, cereal, frozen pies... all gone. The herd fed its fear, swallowing sugar like last rites, stockpiling inflammation in the name of preparedness.

But the vampire did not rush. He did not kneel at the altar of flour. He fasted. He waited. His blood did not tremble.

The Plague Walker

He walks through cities of rot without fear. Not because he is undead, but because he is uninfectable. Not because he cannot catch what floats in the breath of the herd, but because his terrain does not invite the guest.

He does not eat sugar. He does not worship seed oil. He does not sleep drugged or eat by clock or cue. He is fasted, fed on flesh, and forged by fire. And when the world fell into fear, he did not cough. He fed once, deeply, and waited.

His blood didn't fear... it remembered.

The Sick Soil

The world prepared to fight a virus, but it never asked why the virus found such fertile ground. The headlines screamed about transmission. But few dared ask: What made us so easy to infect? It wasn't the air. It was the flesh.

The greatest predictor of severe outcomes from COVID-19 wasn't exposure. It was terrain.

Metabolic syndrome, insulin resistance, obesity, hypertension, fatty liver, was the single strongest risk factor for hospitalization and death[1]. Inflammation, not infection, became the death sentence.

And that terrain wasn't born overnight. It was built over decades, fed by seed oil, sugar, and fear. High insulin is viral Viagra. Seed oils are cytokine kindling. Modern humans weren't infected... they were metabolically self-immolating.

The Carbohydrate Comorbidity

To fear the germ while fueling it is the great modern madness. Every infected cell becomes a biochemical factory, and the primary fuel is glucose. Viral replication accelerates in high-insulin, high-glucose environments[2]. Blood glucose above 140 mg/dL has been shown to increase viral replication by 300 percent in human airways[3]. Sugar doesn't just feed the host. It feeds the invader.

And when the shelves emptied in March of 2020, what disappeared? Rice. Bread. Sugar. Cereal. Rice shelves emptied while viral loads filled. We did not prepare with nutrition. We prepared with the carbohydrates of our childhood grave.

Dr. Benjamin Bikman, a leader in insulin research, called insulin resistance "the defining feature of COVID susceptibility." [4] Dr. Aseem Malhotra called it "the pandemic beneath the pandemic." [5] A 2023 *Lancet* study of over 1.2 million patients[6] proved it: HbA1c above 5.7 percent resulted in a 4.2 times higher COVID mortality. The virus didn't discriminate, but metabolic dysfunction did.

But the carnivore had already cleaned house. Low insulin. Low triglycerides. Low visceral fat. No candy in the bloodstream. No buffet for the breath-born enemy.

The vampire was already in ketosis[7].

Seed Oil Sabotage: The Fire Inside

When the body is inflamed, immunity collapses. Cytokine storms, once a rare medical term, became a household fear. But what primed the storm?

The answer was in the pantry. Seed oils, rich in linoleic acid, are cellular saboteurs. They don't just inflame; they alter mitochondrial function. They embed into membranes like rust on iron. They force cells to breathe through sludge.

And when viral chaos enters a linoleic-rich host, it finds firewood soaked in gasoline. Seed oils are liquid treason, pumping linoleic acid into membranes like saboteurs drilling holes in a ship's hull.

Dr. Paul Mason warned us. But the deeper science now confirms it. Nørgaard's 2023 study showed that linoleic acid exposure after viral challenge elevated IL-6 and TNF-α by over 400 percent[8].

Carnivores carry none of it. No oils. No ultra-processing. No oxidized fats. Their cells are not kindling. They are gilded armor, forged in ancestral fire. Liver wasn't his meal. It was biological chainmail.

Micronutrient Immunity: Flesh as Pharmacy

There is no immune system. There is only an immune state. And it is forged, or failed, in the kitchen. Every immune cell is built from the raw materials we eat, and most modern diets are starved of what immunity needs:

- **Zinc**: Required for T-cell formation and viral inhibition[9]
- **Vitamin D3**: Modulates over 2,000 genes, including those governing infection response[10]
- **Selenium**: Critical for glutathione and antiviral protection
- **Retinol (Vitamin A)**: Shapes mucosal defense and innate immunity

- **Iron**: Powers macrophages, the predator cells of the immune fleet

Liver isn't just food. It's a biological cheat code. 3oz delivers:

- **27,000 IU** Vitamin A (retinol, not beta-carotene)
- **4.7 mg** heme iron
- **300 percent** RDA Copper
- **80 percent** RDA Selenium[11]

These nutrients aren't in gummy vitamins. They're in blood. Fat. Organs. Flesh. The carnivore carries them daily. The plant-based eater does not. The vampire doesn't sip smoothies. He drinks the only elixir that ever-defended life.

The infected herd ate its own funeral feast, grain stockpiles becoming glucose coffins.

The Fast That Protects

There is a silence in the body that heals. Fasting is not starvation. It is the ancestral software of survival. It activates autophagy, the recycling of broken cells and viral debris. It enhances mitochondrial repair. It stimulates the birth of new immune cells[12].

This is not theory. This is immunomctabolism. Carnivores don't need to 'start a fast.' They live there. OMAD. Deep ketosis. A metabolism that doesn't flinch when food disappears. Ancient tribes understood this intuitively.

During sickness, they withdrew. They did not eat. They waited.

The Tsimane hunter-gatherers, during illness, fasted, recovering three times faster than neighboring grain-eating farmers[13]. Because the body knew… to fight the invisible, become metabolically invisible.

The vampire does not graze. He fasts. He heals. He endures.

The Girl in the Smoke

She watched them from her window. Faces lit blue by phones. Pantries swollen with pasta. The air outside was quiet, but inside every home was noise: newsfeed, sugar, fear.

Her companion said little. That night, he salted a thick slice of liver and set it by the fire. "Are you afraid?" she asked. He smiled. "Of what?" She did not answer. She hadn't seen a carrot in weeks. There were no biscuits. No rice. No bread. Only fat. Salt. Meat. And silence.

The searing liver delivered **18,000 IU** of retinol to fortify her lungs, **15 mg** zinc to arm her NK cells, **120 mcg** selenium to ignite glutathione.

When the ambulance screamed past, the smell of liver filled the room, iron and defiance against the scent of sterile panic. She watched again. Her breath calm. Her hunger sharp. He nodded once. "We wait." And they did.

The Doctor Who Did Not Obey

He was retired. Quiet. Once respected. They told him to stay home. So, he did. And he cooked liver. They told him to eat cereal. He threw it away. They told him to mask, to swab, to fear. He nodded politely and went for a walk.

He fasted every third day. Took no pills. Slept when the sun set. His D3 level: **68 ng/mL**. His zinc: **140 mcg/dL**. His fasted blood glucose: **74 mg/dL**.

When he caught it, it lasted one night. Fever, then sleep. Then nothing. His neighbor died. His nephew lost his breath. But he? He stirred his bone broth, steam curling like incense. Outside, sirens wept. Inside, his cells sang the old songs of survival.

The Germ, the Gospel, and the Flame

This chapter is not about COVID. It is about memory. The immune system is not a defense force. It is a memory palace, one built cell by cell, by the foods we choose and the fires we honor.

You were told to fear the germ. But you were never told to fear the terrain that welcomes it. You were told to spray surfaces. Not to strip your pantry. To take drugs. Not to take dominion over your cells.

But the vampire does not kneel. He fasts. He feeds once, deeply. He walks through sickness as myth, not because he is fantasy, but because he is metabolically sovereign.

This is not immunity. This is metabolic sovereignty, your exiled birthright.

Let the herd cough. Your cells sing the old songs of immunity, ketone-fueled, cholesterol-armored, unbroken since the steppes.

Chapter 26

The Hollowing - Hunger Drugs and the Disappearing Woman

Metabolic vanishing and how hunger drugs erase women's bodies

They didn't want to be powerful. They wanted to be small. They traded the strength of flesh for the silence of the scale. They told themselves they were taking control, but their bones whispered otherwise. The marrow knew.

There is a new hunger on the rise, manufactured, not earned. A hunger not for meat, not even for thinness, but for erasure. Women no longer fast to grow wise or holy. They vanish in syringes, in hashtags, in fluorescent waiting rooms lined with pill-bright promises.

They call it progress. I call it the hollowing.

Modern Sorcery

The spell has a name. Several, in fact: semaglutide, liraglutide, dulaglutide. Branded as Ozempic, Wegovy, Mounjaro. Once prescribed for diabetes, these GLP-1 agonists are now the talismans of modern body modification, syringes of surrender disguised as self-care.

GLP-1 drugs are metabolic vampirism. They siphon muscle, bone, and fertility to feed pharmaceutical profits.

But unlike the vampire who honors hunger, these drugs execrate appetite, the soul's biological compass.

While these drugs provide therapeutic relief for conditions like type 2 diabetes and PCOS, their cosmetic repurposing exploits hunger, fear, and insecurity. They work by mimicking a gut hormone that slows gastric emptying and suppresses appetite. But here's the truth no influencer whispers: "You're not eating less because you're full. You're eating less because your brain thinks you're ill." [1]

These drugs induce a biochemical famine. They hijack your metabolic feedback loops, deaden your hunger cues, and leave your body cannibalizing itself. Muscle vanishes. Bone thins. Libido dims. Hormones fall silent. In some, suicidal ideation has emerged, prompting ongoing investigation.[10]

And still, they smile for selfies with sunken cheeks and captioned thigh gaps.

The Hollowing

Let's speak plainly. These drugs do not sculpt you. They dissolve you. This is not weight loss. It is biological strip-mining. Muscle becomes slurry. Bone becomes dust. Wombs become silent catacombs.

1. Bone Loss: GLP-1 agonists impair osteoblast activity, the very cells responsible for building bone. [2] Studies show that weight loss from these drugs often includes a

5.7% annual reduction in spinal bone mineral density in women, compared to 0.9% in untreated controls. [3] This rate is more severe than menopausal decline.

They did not become beautiful. They became brittle.

2. Muscle Wasting: Up to 20–30% of weight lost on GLP-1 drugs is lean mass, [4] with accelerated loss, up to 200% faster, when combined with low-protein diets. Organs shrink. Heart, liver, and muscle. Even the uterus contracts. This isn't optimization. It's atrophy.

3. Nutrient Deficiency: Nausea, vomiting, and delayed digestion impair absorption of key nutrients. Heme iron absorption declines by 37%. [5] Zinc intake drops by 50%. Protein assimilation falters. These are the very nutrients a carnivore diet restores with precision, especially from red meat, liver, marrow, and salt.

4. Fertility Fallout: GLP-1 drugs disrupt the hypothalamic-pituitary-gonadal axis.[6] Ovulation becomes irregular or ceases entirely. Amenorrhea affects up to 22% of users, compared to 4% in placebo groups.[7] Some stop menstruating altogether, often lauded as a "bonus" of thinness. But this is not liberation. This is metabolic shutdown. Primate studies show arrested ovarian follicles.

A carnivore way of eating, in contrast, feeds the body into balance. Cholesterol becomes the substrate for sex hormones. Organs are nourished, not diminished. Meat reawakens the cycles that starvation silences.

The Metaphor

Hunger is not a flaw. It is fire. It is memory.

The vampire does not flee hunger. He honors it. He sharpens his teeth to meet it. Hunger tells him he's alive. Hunger is the signal that the body still believes in its own worth.

The modern woman has been taught that hunger is disobedience. And so, she takes the shot. Not to feel full, but to feel nothing. This is not vampirism. This is necromancy. A pharmaceutically induced death state where appetite, our deepest ancestral compass, is numbed.

The vampire remembers a time when hunger forged warriors. Now it forges patients. Even fangs require calcium. So do your bones.

Cultural Critique

Pharmaceutical companies know exactly what they're doing. Their campaigns target women with surgical precision: "Take control of your weight."; "A new you."; "Power in a pen." But it's not power they're selling. It's disappearance.

Physicians often receive bonuses or incentives for prescribing these drugs.[8] In 2023 alone, Novo Nordisk paid over 57 U.S. doctors more than $100,000 each to promote Wegovy and Saxenda. One doctor earned $1.4

million.[8] In states like Vermont where gift bans exist, diabetes drug costs fell 3–8%.[8]

Meanwhile, the monthly cost of Wegovy in the U.S. is $1,349. In the UK and Germany, it's $92.[9] Senator Sanders called it plainly: "The U.S. is Novo Nordisk's cash cow."[9]

Influence tactics include:

- Massive speaking fees to prescribers, with some earning seven figures
- Viral social media campaigns, such as over 400 million TikTok views for #Ozempic
- Nutritional misinformation that encourages low-protein diets, which in turn amplifies muscle loss by up to 200%

Girls lose their periods, their hunger, their will to take up space. Doctors get paid. Pharma wins.

Social Media Sorcery

Ozempic face. TikTok jawlines. Hollow cheekbones trending like lipstick shades. These are not signs of health. They are signs of systemic catabolism. Facial collapse from masseter muscle atrophy has now been clinically documented.[11]

Smallness has become a virtue. Hunger, a pathology. To eat meat is considered grotesque. To eat nothing is considered grace. You used to be told to take up space.

Now you're told to subtract yourself. But in the world of the carnivore, we do not subtract. We devour.

The Woman Who Faded

She started with portion control. Then intermittent fasting. Then shakes. Then syringes.

At first, the compliments poured in. "You look amazing." "What's your secret?" "You're glowing." (She wasn't, perhaps it was concealer.)

She missed her period. Her libido withered. Her bones ached in winter. Still, the praise kept coming.

But one night, under a weak moon, something inside her snapped. It wasn't rebellion. It was remembrance. She walked barefoot to the woods. Dug her fingers into the dirt. Found a rabbit carcass, half-eaten by a fox. She knelt. She wept. And then, she ate.

She roasted meat on sticks. She cracked bones with stones. She licked the liver's warm iron. A wolf howled. Her spine straightened. Her breath thickened. Her hunger returned. So did her strength. So did her cycle. So did her voice.

She never counted calories again. She counted fires. She counted red suns. She wore a necklace of bone and bark and blood. And when she passed other fading women, she whispered: "You were not meant to vanish. You were meant to burn."

Resurrection

There is another path. Eat fat, not fear. Meat restores what needles erase. It feeds the bones. Fuels the hormones. Fortifies the will. While Semaglutide dissolves muscle, carnivore eating rebuilds it. For example:

- Bone broth glycine increases osteoblast activity by 200%
- Heme iron reverses amenorrhea in 86% of women[12]
- Dietary cholesterol converts to pregnenolone, restoring progesterone levels

The carnivore way is not a trend. It is a return. To fire. To fang. To flesh. To the ritual of satiety. Hunger is the ancestral drumbeat. Meat is the anti-needle. Your body is not a disposal problem. It is a sacred fire demanding fuel.

This chapter does not critique weight management. It critiques disappearance for profit. Health exists at every size, but not when pharma profits from vanishing women.

You were not designed for scarcity. You were designed for strength. Red meat is not rebellion. It is remembrance. A remembering of bone, blood, and becoming.

Reclamation Checklist

- Prioritize bone broth and connective tissue for collagen
- Eat fatty ruminant meat daily for hormonal support
- Track protein intake ($\geq$1g per pound lean mass)

- Monitor cycle health, mood, and sleep as metabolic markers
- Lift heavy things; muscle is medicine
- Ditch scales; build strength instead

Better to be full of blood than full of lies. Hunger is not your enemy. It is your inheritance.

Chapter 27

Gut Healing & Immune Reset

The gut is not just a tube. It is a temple. A torch. A truth-teller beneath the skin.

The Wound Within

The modern gut is not a digestive organ. It is a wounded battlefield. A battlefield lined with bandages, bloated with betrayal, inflamed with the residue of seed oils and sterile bread.

Once, the gut was a forge. It sealed what it did not trust. It burned what it did not need. It moved with the rhythm of hunger and the discipline of kill. But now it leaks. Wheat and seed oils drive zonulin into overexpression. Tight junctions unzip like traitorous gates. Lipopolysaccharides march into blood, saboteurs disguised as nutrients[1].

And the body retaliates. LPS binds to immune sentries like TLR4, screaming "invader." The body fires on its own, confusing the echo of wheat for the echo of self[2]. Psoriasis. IBS. Eczema. Brain fog. Celiac. MCAS. Autoimmunity of a thousand names, each a reflection of one wound. A fire that has turned inward.

The Crypt and the Graveyard

The vampire's gut does not leak. It is sealed like a crypt: acidic, disciplined, clean. There is no garden in it. No mulch, no fiber, no rot. It remembers what it is: a chamber of fire, not fermentation. A distiller of blood, not a compost bin for kale.

The modern gut is a graveyard: domesticated, sluggish, overgrown with bacteria that never belonged. The cult of fiber feeds this decay. "Feed your microbiome," they chant. But what if your ancestral microbiome was forged on marrow, not mulch? On collagen, not cellulose?

Hunter guts, Inuit, Maasai, Mongol, thrived on raw meat, fermented blood, and bone broth. No salads. No sourdough. No prebiotics. Yet no disease. No cavities. No Crohn's[3]. When meat flowed, their guts abandoned fiber. When famine came, a root or tuber might pass through, tolerated, never glorified[4].

Some meat-fed microbes do not ferment. They fight. They release bacteriocins, slaughtering the sugar-fed rot. Butyrate becomes their ceasefire, a mucosal mender[5].

The Neolithic gut is not evolution. It is disconnection. A metabolic divorce from ancestral symbiosis.

The vampire remembers. And he does not rot.

Asa and the Firekeeper

The boy was seven when the pain began. They called it IBS. Then leaky gut. Then autoimmune enterocolitis. Doctors tried formulas. Antibiotics. Fiber shakes. But his belly stayed swollen. His sleep stayed shallow. His skin stayed grey.

At night he cried for fire. But he was given oat milk. He begged for marrow. But he was prescribed sedatives.

Until the old woman came. She said nothing at first. Only watched. Then she boiled bones for 48 hours and salted them with her own hands. She fasted with the boy. Taught him to sip broth before sunrise. Then raw liver, pressed between his teeth. Then fat. Then silence. She added raw egg yolks to the broth. IgY immunoglobulins, ancient antibodies, binding the lectins his zonulin had once welcomed[6].

On the sixth night, Asa's bile turned thick and dark, burning biofilm like fire on old skin. The *Enterococcus faecalis* that had colonized his ileum died screaming in bile acids[7].

By the ninth night, his bowels did not cramp. On the twelfth, his skin turned pink with blood. On the fifteenth, he stood without trembling. He did not ask for cereal again.

Before leaving, the woman whispered one thing in his ear: "Do not feed the wound. Feed the fire."

And Asa, the boy they had once called fragile, became the one who could walk through winter without a coat. They said his gut had healed. But Asa knew the truth. His gut had remembered.

The Three Flames of Immunity

Your gut was once a napalm moat. Now it's a damp match. To rebuild it, you must relight your three flames:

1. **Acidic Inferno**: Your stomach once held a pH below 1.5. Pathogens dissolved before they reached the blood.
2. **Bile Torch**: Secondary bile acids like deoxycholate incinerated invaders[8]. Bile that now stagnates must burn again.
3. **Mucosal Magma**: Butyrate from meat-fed microbes fuels the regeneration of mucin, a living fire curtain[9].

Modern guts lack fire. Yours will not.

The Second Brain

Before you had a face, you had a gut. In the womb, the enteric nervous system forms first. A neural lattice of over 100 million neurons, mirroring the spinal cord, pulsing with ancient signal[10].

Long before the first bite, the gut was already thinking. It was already listening. This is why we say: "I have a gut feeling."; "My gut says no."; "I knew it in my belly."

Because you did. The gut is not just digestive. It is cognitive. Hormonal. Immunological. It is your oldest brain, buried beneath breath.

The vagus nerve ferries fire between the belly and the skull, mood, memory, hunger, immunity. Serotonin. Dopamine. GABA. All shaped, not just in the brain, but in the gut[11].

Your gut produces 90% of your serotonin, but grain-fed microbes hold it hostage until you pay their sugar ransom[12]. Feed the gut poison, and the mind forgets. Feed the gut marrow, and the fire returns.

The vampire does not separate instinct from digestion. He knows his gut is an oracle, not a garbage chute. And he listens.

Resurrection by Meat

When some try the carnivore diet, they do it wrong. Eat only chicken and minced beef. No liver. No fat. No marrow. Scorching scurvy-starved bodies[13].

Raw meat contains vitamin C. Fifteen milligrams per pound. It is enough, if you do not fear the blood[14]. Cook it to death, and the C dies with it. But eat it rare, salted, reverently, and the wound stays shut.

Marrow lines the gut with ancestral balm. Fat soothes the fire. Liver tightens the junctions[15]. Fasting silences the microbial mutiny.

Carnivore is not a diet. It is terrain therapy. It is the closing of the gates. Zonulin retreats. LPS fades. The immune system no longer misfires. The wound becomes a wall. The wall becomes a forge. And in that forge, something sacred returns.

I Do Not Feed the Rot

I do not feed the bacteria that never belonged. I do not fiber my gut with poisons wrapped in green. I chew fat because it seals the wall. I eat liver because it remembers the breach. I drink broth because it carries fire into every fold. I fast so that the fire may speak. I eat marrow so that the forge may stay lit.

You fed your gut kale. I fed mine blood. You called it inflammation. I called it forgetting. You called it autoimmunity. I called it betrayal.

But now you remember. Because the hunger was not in your mouth. It was in your belly. Where your ancestors once burned. Where the wolves once hunted. Where the vampire still kneels before the kill.

The Firekeeper's Protocol

The Gut Reset Rite:

1. Fast for 24 hours. Only water plus 2g sodium chloride, activates chloride channels for HCl.
2. Break the fast with marrow broth. Sip slowly.

3. Eat raw liver, one bite. Do not chew with fear. Chew with fire.
4. Walk barefoot at dawn. Grounding reduces TNF-α by 37%[16].
5. Repeat for seven days. On the eighth, eat only meat and fat.
6. On the ninth, write a name: the one you gave your sickness. Burn it with tallox flame. Let the lipid fire erase what plant-fed memory could not.

This is not a cleanse. This is remembrance. This is the sealing of the crypt. The rekindling of the fire. This is gut resurrection. And it begins with blood.

Chapter 28

The Cell That Forgot

Cancer, Metabolic Sovereignty, and the Vampire Who Would Not Rot

The Flesh That Burns Too Soon

The body is not meant to rot from within. Decay was supposed to come later, after the final breath, after the burial flame, after the predator's bones were returned to the soil. But now, it begins early. In silence. In flesh that forgets the code.

There is a betrayal that cuts deeper than the fang. A cell once loyal, once governed by the rhythms of hunger, fire, and death, breaks the pact. It multiplies without reason. It refuses the signal to die. It grows where no growth was asked for. This is not life. This is 'unlife', a cruel parody of the vampire myth. The cancer cell does not die because it forgets.

The vampire lives beyond time because he remembers. The vampire fasts. The cancer cell feeds. The vampire becomes stronger with age. The cancer cell weakens everything around it. One is ancient, sovereign, disciplined. The other is modern, chaotic, wild in the worst way.

You were designed to burn clean: grow when needed, stop when full, die when called. This is the law of the predator. And the law of the cell. Mitochondria are the keepers of this law. When they falter, the code unravels.

But something has happened. And no one wants to say it. The sweet blood, the constant eating, the endless insulin. It has created a terrain not of life, but of unregulated growth. The body, soaked in sugar, becomes a garden for death. A mutiny of fuel. A starvation amidst plenty.

We don't call it that. We give it names. Breast. Colon. Brain. Skin. But beneath the Latin and the lineage, it's all the same thing: A broken rhythm. A betrayal of fire.

Cancer is not a monster. It is the memory of the monster we fed. And so, we fight it, with blades and beams, with chemo and prayers. But rarely do we ask the deeper question: Why does the body forget? Why does the cell rebel? Why does the flesh, in a world of abundance, choose to self-destruct?

The vampire does not ask these questions. He already knows. He knows that the modern human is overfed and undernourished. He knows that glucose is not just fuel, it is signal. He knows that to eat sugar without restraint is not pleasure, it is programming. He remembers a time when hunger was holy. When the kill restored the code. When flesh was the feast, and fire, the purifier.

Cancer cannot thrive in that memory. It requires sweetness. It requires forgetfulness. It requires you to ignore the ancient voice that says: Stop eating. Wait. Burn clean. The vampire obeys this voice. The modern human drowns it in breakfast.

And so, the cell forgets.

Warburg's Flame

Warburg found this forgetting in the breath of cells. In 1924, the German physiologist peered into tumors and discovered something strange. Cancer cells consumed enormous amounts of glucose, even in the presence of oxygen. Where healthy cells used oxygen to fuel mitochondrial respiration, cancer cells bypassed that path. They chose a more primitive process: aerobic glycolysis, fermenting sugar into lactate, even with oxygen available[1].

Warburg believed this was not a symptom. It was the cause: "Cancer, above all other diseases, has countless secondary causes. But, even for cancer, there is only one prime cause. The replacement of the respiration of oxygen in normal body cells by a fermentation of sugar." [Otto Warburg, 1966 Nobel Lecture][2]. This became known as the Warburg Effect.

Cancer is not just a genetic disease. It is a metabolic one. A rebellion of the mitochondria. A cell so starved of breath; it drowns in sugar. Warburg uncovered cancer's dirty secret: tumors ferment like yeast in a sugar vat while mitochondria suffocate.

Seyfried's work shows mitochondrial damage unlocks genetic chaos, like rust crumbling a lock before the thieves enter[3]. Vasan's 2023 study confirms this. Glycolysis-derived reactive oxygen species drive over 60% of oncogenic mutations[4].

And when the mitochondria collapse, they don't just forget how to breathe. They lose their shape. Cristae degenerates. Apoptosis fails[5].

But then came the gene revolution, the Human Genome Project, the pharmaceutical gold rush. Warburg's flame was entombed in genetic dogma.

But not from the shadows. His work returned, resurrected by researchers who now see the terrain collapses before the genome mutates. Because if the soil matters more than the seed, then cancer is not about fate. It's about fuel. And terrain. And flame.

The Terrain Theory Reborn

This was the forgotten wisdom of Antoine Béchamp, a 19th-century rival to Louis Pasteur. While Pasteur insisted that germs caused disease, Béchamp whispered that terrain determines what grows. "Le terrain est tout!" [The terrain is everything!]

His cry was drowned by germ theory. But today, cancer metabolism proves him right. Cancer is not an invader. It is an opportunist. A scavenger of the metabolic wasteland. High glucose. High insulin. Chronic inflammation. Impaired autophagy. These are not symptoms of cancer. They are the soil that feeds it.

And this is why the vampire does not rot. He does not graze. He feasts and fasts. He lives in precision, glucose low, insulin flat, ketones sharp.

Germ theory won the war. But the terrain is winning the science.

Hunger as Healing

WARNING: Metabolic therapy supports conventional cancer care. It is not a replacement. Always work with your oncology team. Also NOTE: low-glucose strategies may not apply to hematologic cancers (leukemia, lymphoma) where immune function is glucose-dependent. Context is king.

The vampire's oldest tactic. Fasting is terrain warfare. It clears debris, restores rhythm, and exposes the enemy. When the body goes without food, something ancient awakens. Autophagy, the Greek for "self-eating," is not destruction. It is dismantling with purpose. It recycles broken proteins and devours damaged mitochondria, scavengers turned traitors if left unchecked[6]. Insulin falls. Fire returns. Mitochondria remember. Ketones rise, not just as fuel, but as messengers. They silence inflammation and inhibit HDACs, releasing tumor-suppressor genes long silenced by metabolic noise[7-8]. They also downregulate HIF-1α, starving tumors of new blood supply[9].

Clinical trials show glioblastoma patients on ketogenic protocols live significantly longer, 11.2 vs 7.8 months, when combined with standard care[10]. Other studies reveal that fasting and low-carb nutrition reduce chemotherapy side effects and improve recovery[11]. Valter Longo's fasting-mimicking diet shows enhanced synergy with chemo and reduced toxicity[12]. De Groot's work reveals that fasting preserves over 20 billion lymphocytes from chemotherapy damage[13].

This is not starvation. It is strategy. And the vampire knows it well.

The Butcher's Daughter

They told her to eat. She had lost her hair, her strength, her sleep, but the nurses still pushed the tray forward. Pudding. Toast. Orange juice. A smile. "You need energy," they said.

She looked at the tray as if it were poison. Not because she thought meat would cure her. Not because she had read about mitochondria. But because somewhere in her marrow, she remembered. She remembered her grandfather's fasts. The silence. The broth. The ritual. They had called her the butcher's daughter. As if the fire might pass through the blood.

She didn't want to die with sugar on her breath. So, she refused the tray. She asked for broth. Salt. Meat, if they had it. Liver, if they dared. They didn't. But her sister smuggled it in. Wrapped in foil. Still warm from a flame. It was veal liver, high in vitamin K2. It smelled of iron and earth, like wet soil after rain. Each bite was a rite.

Matrix Gla proteins stirred. Metastasis calcification was denied.

She didn't expect to live forever. She just didn't want to rot sweetly. The other women whispered behind the curtain. The cloying sweetness of Ensure on their breath. She didn't judge them. She just chose another way. They called her 'the liver rebel', the woman who chose mitochondrial fidelity over institutional sucrose.

Weeks passed. No miracle came. But neither did collapse. Her bloodwork stabilized. Her strength held. And when her doctor asked what she was doing, she said: "I'm not feeding it."

This is not a story of survival. It is a story of sovereignty. And the body remembers that. Years later, the nurses still whispered her name. She was the one who refused to rot sweetly.

The Vampire Doesn't Rot

Decay is not fate. It is metabolic amnesia. The human body does not erupt. It ferments. It swells. It slides. But the vampire does not rot. Not because he is blessed. But because he remembers. He remembers when to fast. When to feast. When to wait.

The vampire's secret isn't immortality. It's fidelity to rhythm. Feast after the hunt. Fast beneath snow. Burn at the moon's command. Feast. Fast. Burn. Repeat. His mitochondria do not panic. They remember how to burn.

A Sacred Warning

This chapter is not a miracle. It promises no cure, only sovereignty in the fire. Cancer is not just mutation. It is terrain collapse. And terrain can be remembered.

Not all cancers are alike. But many share the same terrain, sugar, swelling, and silence. To fast is to break that silence. To eat flesh is to sharpen the edge. To wait is to burn clean.

You may burn out... but you will not fall soft. You will not rot sweetly. You will burn. Like the vampire. In rhythm. In fire. In memory.

Feed your mitochondria, not your mutations. Fast your insulin, not your hope. Burn clean. Remember. The vampire does.

Chapter 29

The Undrugged Mind

He who does not sedate his blood remembers everything.

The White-Pill Priesthood

The sacraments are stamped with lot numbers. The altar is your bedside drawer. The rite: a white pill swallowed with filtered water and a touch of morning fear.

Medicine used to mean healing. Now it means management. Regulation. Sedation. We do not cure. We suppress. We dampen. We medicate.

This is not a polemic against medicine. It is a requiem for what medicine used to be: a call to wholeness. Today's prescriptions are not rooted in reverence, but in revenue. The protocol is not sacred, it is sponsored. The guidelines come not from shamans, but from shareholders. Their miracles come with 47 pages of side effects.

A pill is not just a molecule. It is a signal. A signal that says: your body is wrong; your chemistry must comply. It tells you: don't feel; don't fast; don't fight. It promises that you can stay domesticated and to just take this.

But something in you remembers. The hunger. The heat. The hurt that healed through its own fire.

Biological Sovereignty

You were not born with a prescription in your hand. You were born with the ability to fast. To flare. To recover. You were born for cortisol that crests with the dawn, not pills that flatten it. You were born for dopamine that drips from the hunt, not serotonin sold by the capsule. You were born with metabolic rhythm, not chemical override.

The vampire never lost this memory. He does not ask for healing, because he never agreed to be sick. To outsource your biology is to abandon your kingdom.

They gave you pills because they stole your hunt. They replaced the predator with the protocol. They medicated your instincts and called it progress.

Golden Blood: The Cholesterol Lie

Cholesterol is not the villain. It is the crown. It is golden blood: the scaffold of your synapses, the architect of your hormones, the repairman of your vessels. It is the elixir from which you synthesize sex, sunlight, and sanity. Your liver produces 80 percent of it. The enemy was never cholesterol. It was oxidation.

Cholesterol only becomes a villain when inflamed, scorched by seed oils, glycated by sugar. In a body burning clean, it is liquid gold. Cholesterol sulfate, abundant in grass-fed meat, repels pathogens while stabilizing cell membranes. Statins strip this armor.

Yet this vital molecule was recast as a killer, not because of truth, but because of patents. You cannot patent ribeye. You can patent a statin.

Statins: The Great Sedation

Statins do not heal. They silence. They induce insulin resistance, the very driver of diabetic pathology[1]. They deplete CoQ10 by up to 51 percent, especially in cardiac tissue[2]. They elevate dementia risk by accelerating hippocampal atrophy by over 30 percent[3]. They suppress LDL, the same lipoprotein that binds and neutralizes endotoxins[4].

LDL is not a clog. It is a shield. It protects against infection, binds bacterial toxins, and orchestrates tissue repair[5]. Kruth (2023) showed that LDL binds lipopolysaccharides five times more effectively than antibiotics[6].

Seed oils oxidize LDL[7], turning shield into shrapnel. Mason (2024) demonstrated that seed oil peroxides glycate LDL eight times faster than glucose[8]. Ruminant fats, by contrast, armor it.

Statins rarely heal the root cause. They are biological silencers. For the 1 percent with familial hypercholesterolemia, they may be a necessary compromise. But never the first resort.

Yes, statins may add years to a life already broken by metabolic chaos. But what if we prevented the chaos instead? Sedating symptoms is not healing. It is biological betrayal. The vampire tastes statins in your blood... and retches gold.

The Village That Took the Pill and Forgot the Kill

They lived at the edge of the forest, where wolves once sang and children once fasted. No one starved. No one hunted. No one remembered how.

The elders gathered at dawn, swallowing beige disks with filtered water, like swallows pecking gravel. They called it "wellness," as if surrender had a new name.

The children grew soft. The venison turned to porridge in their mouths. Muscle became murmured complaint. Silence became symptom. No one died of heart disease. But they no longer knew what a heart was for.

And then, one winter, the pills ran out. No one knew how to butcher. No one knew how to wait. The cold remembered them, but they'd forgotten how to shiver.

Long before Lipitor, pre-statin Icelanders had LDL levels over 180 mg/dL and heart disease rates under 3 percent[9]. Their secret? Fermented shark, lamb fat, and no fear of fat.

Cholesterol: Not a Threat, A Throne

High cholesterol is not a flaw. It is a crown of sovereignty, Worn by brains that burn fat, Hormones that howl at the moon, And nerves wrapped in golden myelin. It fuels your brain. Builds your hormones. Protects your nerves. LDL defends against pathogens[5]. HDL scavenges waste. Together, they form a circulatory covenant.

The truly sick often have the lowest cholesterol. The dying lose their gold first. You were taught to fear what your ancestors honored. But the vampire remembers.

Medicine Wasn't Always This

There were once doctors who fasted with the sick. Who prescribed liver, not Lunesta. Who understood that fever was a furnace of healing, not something to be extinguished like an alarm.

In every village, there was one who carried bone knives and knew the names of hunger. They whispered rituals, not risk factors. They trusted the kill more than the cure. That was medicine.

What we have now is managed decline. Remember Hippocrates', "let food be thy medicine." Remember Weston Price and his X-factor butter oil. Remember Semmelweis and the revolt of clean hands.

The Mind That Refused the Spell

The vampire does not take pills. Because his mind is not broken. It is undrugged. Truth is not a chemical. It is a frequency, the hum of mitochondria burning fat, the resonance of a body remembering fire.

Your mind was never meant to be medicated into meekness. It was meant to ache. To burn. To rebuild. I do not scorn those who take pills. I mourn those never offered fire.

The Vampiric Monologue

You are not sick. You are drugged. Your hunger is not a disorder. Your grief is not an error code. It is gravity.

They diagnosed your hunger as pathology. I diagnose their prescriptions as epitaphs. They broke your rituals and replaced them with regimens. They fear your silence, because it is where the truth begins.

I do not ask for healing, because I never agreed to be sick. The vampire's 'pale immortality' is preserved in cholesterol-rich tissue. Slavic graves show no atherosclerosis ... only the echo of fat-burning fire.

Invocation: Reclaiming Fire

To reclaim your sovereignty:

- Eat like an apex, not an algorithm

- Salt your meat like a rebel salts the earth of empires
- Fast until clarity bites back
- Feast until fear forgets you
- Move when the sun stalks or the moon bleeds, not when a screen flickers
- Trust the ache
- Remember the hunt

The body is not broken. It was meant to burn through lies.

The Undrugged Protocol

You were not born to be sedated. You were born to be sovereign. Begin here:

- Fasting is firmware ritual. Each hour resets the ancestral signal: quieting noise, refining memory, sharpening truth. Fasting insulin should fall below 3 µIU/mL.
- Ketosis is a cognitive torch. The brain feeds on ketones. Memory strengthens. Inflammation falls silent. Maalouf et al. (2009) showed ketone metabolism shields neurons from toxic assault[10]. Kashiwaya (2023) revealed ketones increase hippocampal mitochondrial biogenesis by over 200 percent[11]. Target ketones: 0.5 to 3.0 mM.
- Cholesterol is cellular armor. It fortifies every membrane, every synapse. It's not the enemy; it's your inner goldsmith. LDL Pattern A, large and fluffy, is

protective. HDL is the scavenger and repair agent. Vitamin D should rise above 50 ng/mL.

- Animal fats are ancestral language. They whisper fertility, clarity, truth to your cells, the same lipids that lit the lamps of Lascaux. They don't sedate. They awaken.

- Movement is medicine. Not treadmills, but torque. Not burnout, but blood. The kind that makes your mitochondria sing in ketone minor.

- Sunlight is signal. Not filtered. Not feared. Real light. On real skin. Telling your pineal gland the truth of the hour.

If you are taking pills now, hear this: Sovereignty begins not in defiance, but in curiosity. Ask: What made my blood so loud they had to silence it? Ask: Who profits when golden blood is recast as poison? Who wins when steak is swapped for statins?

This is not a condemnation of all medicine. Emergency medicine saves lives. This chapter critiques preventive care corrupted by profit, not the hands that pull us from the fire.

Chapter 30

The Bloodline - The Forgotten Lineage of the Flesh-Fed

"In a time of deceit, telling the truth is a revolutionary act."
George Orwell

Metabolic Martyrs: The Heretics Who Preserved Carnivore Truth

They wore lab coats, not capes. They did not hide in shadows or feed on maidens. They walked brightly lit corridors, penned warnings in longhand, and whispered metabolic truths into the rising storm of agricultural industrialism. They were the vampires of the flesh-fed, those who remembered. And one by one, they were hunted.

Some were mocked. Others were sued. A few were exiled from their professions entirely. Not because they were wrong, but because they were early. Because they stood between empire and appetite. Because their science was not for sale. This is their bloodline. This is their truth.

Jean Anthelme Brillat-Savarin (1755–1826)

A gourmand by taste, but a predator by instinct, Brillat-Savarin's famous line wasn't just culinary. It was cellular. In his 1825, Physiologie du Goût, he foresaw what few dared to say: that sugar and starch lay at the root of obesity, and that fat was not to be feared, but revered.[1] He wrote: "Sugar whitens teeth but rots the viscera; fat feeds the fire of life" - a prophecy of insulin resistance before insulin was even discovered.

His warning was not persecuted so much as buried beneath the rising tide of saccharine romance and powdered refinement. As the industrial sugar trade colonized global tastebuds, the philosopher's metabolic truths sank beneath pastry and politesse. His insights drowned in gastronomy, but they live again in every carnivore who eats with intent.

William Banting (1796–1878)

Banting was not a doctor, but a coffin-maker who carried too much flesh to fit.[2] It exploded through England like a musket shot.

Physicians scorned him, of course. The Lancet labeled his success "quackery" and "dangerous enthusiasm."[3] Its editor, Sir James Paget, later revealed to hold shares in Tate & Lyle, a sugar empire whose future depended on the failure of fat.

Banting's crime? Proving sovereignty cost pennies per day. The establishment needed workers weak, hungry for snacks, dependent. But his results couldn't be buried. His name became a verb, to bant, until the grain-and-syrup machine rolled over it, repackaging dietary truth as calorie-counting compliance.

Vilhjalmur Stefansson (1879–1962)

Stefansson lived among the Inuit for years, thriving on their all-meat diet. When he returned, the scientific establishment scoffed, until he offered himself for study. For a year, he and a colleague ate nothing but meat under medical supervision at Bellevue Hospital.[4]

The outcome? Perfect health. No scurvy, no deficiencies.[5] Later research showed that raw meat provides over 15 mg of vitamin C per pound, enough to prevent deficiency entirely.[6] But headlines labeled the experiment "reckless." *JAMA* dismissed it as theatrical. Stefansson's testimony threatened the grain-fortified lie, and so, they ignored him. He didn't starve in the Arctic. He starved for truth in lecture halls funded by General Mills.

Dr. Wilhelm Ebstein (1836–1912)

Ebstein, a renowned internist, argued that obesity stemmed not from fat, but from excessive carbohydrates.[7] In 1882, he proposed a high-fat, low-carb diet - half a century before it became "radical." In 1883, he published a case study showing that 32 obese patients lost over 20 pounds each on a diet of 80 percent fat, with marked improvements in gout.[8]

In Germany, he was accused of promoting dietary elitism and "irresponsible experimentation." Deutsches Ärzteblatt ran a scathing editorial titled "Gegen die Fett-Diät."[9] His legacy was buried beneath subsidized sugar fields. His guidelines disappeared from medical schools. Not disproven. Just inconvenient.

Dr. Frederick Allen (1879–1964)

Before insulin, diabetes was a death sentence. Allen's solution was brutal but effective: a strict meat-based fasting protocol that extended life, often for years.[10]

But Allen couldn't patent fasting. And he had no corporate sponsor. When Eli Lilly introduced insulin, it was profitable, injectable, and infinitely marketable. Allen's work? Not so much.[11] He extended lives without patents. A fatal flaw in Pharma's economy.

Dr. Karl Petrén (1868–1927)

Petrén, working from Lund, Sweden, refined Allen's theories by emphasizing high-fat ketogenic therapy for diabetes. His patients improved.[12] He pioneered a 4:1 fat-to-carb-plus-protein ratio, nearly identical to today's clinical protocols for epilepsy.

But in 1923, insulin's mass production rendered his non-pharmaceutical method obsolete in the eyes of a hungry industry. Eli Lilly's insulin marketing buried his ketogenic protocol. It was not that Petrén failed. It was that he made medicine too simple.

Dr. Wolfgang Lutz (1913–2010)

A man of sharp suits and sharper prose, Lutz published Leben ohne Brot ("Life Without Bread") in 1967, warning of the link between carbohydrate excess and degenerative disease.[13] He was mocked relentlessly, especially by the German nutrition boards.

His diet worked. His patients healed. But textbooks moved on without him, preferring sugar subsidies and cereal endorsements to data. It wasn't science that rejected him. It was policy.

Professor John Yudkin (1910–1995)

Yudkin's 1972 book *Pure, White and Deadly* landed like a stake through Big Sugar's heart.[14] He warned that sugar, not fat, was fueling heart disease, diabetes, and obesity.

They silenced him. The sugar industry paid Harvard scientists to discredit him and elevate Ancel Keys' lipid hypothesis.[15] Yudkin's department was defunded. His research shunned. In 2024, his unpublished manuscript resurfaced, showing a 300 percent rise in liver fat among sugar-fed primates.[16] He was right. And now his ghost stains every sugar-coated guideline with truth.

Dr. Jan Kwaśniewski (1937–2019)

In Communist Poland, Kwaśniewski preached what few dared: high fat, low carb, meat-based living. His "Optimal Diet" healed patients with obesity, epilepsy, and autoimmune disease.[17] By 2023, leaked medical records from Warsaw University showed an 86 percent remission rate in rheumatoid arthritis, compared to 22 percent with conventional immunosuppressants.

But pharmaceutical lobbyists labeled his protocol "dangerous dogma." Polish health boards, under EU pressure, revoked his clinic license.[18] His clinics went underground. His message survived.

Dr. Richard K. Bernstein (b. 1934)

A Type 1 diabetic and former engineer, Bernstein used a home glucometer to experiment on himself. The result? A low-carb protocol that normalized his blood sugar.[19]

The ADA's 1989 Standards of Care excluded low-carb protocols, citing Lilly-funded studies.[20] In a 1991 letter, Eli Lilly allegedly threatened to withdraw funding if the ADA endorsed his approach.[21] Bernstein's book was banned from many clinics. He wasn't excluded for being wrong, but for daring to solve diabetes without selling drugs.

Dr. Herman Taller (1906–1984)

Taller promoted weight loss via safflower oil, believing polyunsaturated fats could reverse metabolic disease. His book *Calories Don't Count* sold millions. But his claims angered the FDA, which accused him of deceptive marketing tied to unregulated supplements.[22]

He wasn't silenced for defending animal fat. He was punished for threatening Procter & Gamble's Crisco empire. They needed a public execution. He was it.

Dr. Blake Donaldson (1890–1966)

Donaldson treated obesity, diabetes, and heart disease at New York's Presbyterian Hospital using an all-meat diet. His patients improved, until the hospital expelled him in 1962, accusing him of "endangering children" with grain-free protocols. His legacy was buried, but the flesh-fed remember.

Mary Enig (1931–2014)

A biochemist and lipid specialist, was among the first to expose the dangers of trans fats while the USDA promoted Crisco. Her work was dismissed as hysteria, her funding blocked. Yet decades later, she was vindicated. Margarine melted. The seed oil empire cracked. Her voice still echoes in every sizzling skillet of tallow.

'The Unnamed Carnivore'

You know him. He carries the bloodline. He walks the night of modernity, devouring misinformation. He does not eat for likes. He does not kneel for moderation. He waits for the kill. He sharpens the truth like a fang.

You will not find him on morning television. You will not hear him from dieticians with sponsors. But if you listen, truly listen, you will hear the hunger. Beneath the silence. Beneath the shame.

These pioneers were metabolic vampires, drinking truth from ancestral veins while industry tried to stake them with subsidies. Like Slavs hiding from grain priests, they preserved forbidden science in blood-stained manuscripts.

You will remember. You will fast. You will feast. The lifeblood of our resistance. They sowed lies in the soil of our silence. Now witness the harvest.

Your plate is the protest. Your hunger, the evidence. The bloodstain is our sacrament. The fast, our communion. The sizzle of fat in the pan, our battle hymn.

__Chapter 31__

The Red Flame

You were never meant to eat quietly.

The Ascension

You've come far. Not just in pages, but in presence. You have not been reading. You have been remembering.

Somewhere between the silence of your first fast and the taste of your first fearless bite, something ancient stirred in you. Not new. Not learned. Remembered.

That is the truth of this journey. It was never about discovery. It was about return.

And I, I did not write these words as a witness. I walked them with you. I bled with you. I burned with you. I am not your coach. I am not your guru. I am what you are becoming: undoped, undrugged, undying. I am the one who remembered before you did. And I stayed behind, not to lead you, but to walk beside you. Until now.

Because now, you don't need me. You are no longer the student. You are the fire.

The Flame Was Always in You

You felt it, didn't you? That flicker at first, when you skipped a meal and realized you didn't die. When you ate steak instead of sadness. When your eyes cleared. When your skin warmed in the sun and something in your blood whispered, "This is what I was made for". That whisper wasn't mine. That was you. The old you. The real you. The one buried under seed oils, cereal boxes, and silence.

You weren't sick. You were silenced. You weren't weak. You were lied to. But you fasted. You killed. You feasted. You remembered.

Somewhere, a boy once walked into the woods and remembered who he was. So did you.

There's an old tale they tried to bury: A village once kept a flame burning in a cave, fed only by animal fat and vigil. "It's savage," said the new priests. "Use oil. It's cleaner." The oil smoked. Eyes watered. Lungs weakened.

One night, a girl slipped into the cave, lit a torch from the old flame, and vanished into the forest. They found her years later, strong, sharp-eyed, surrounded by children who licked fat from their fingers like nectar. Her fire still burns. And it has no barcode.

The Red Pill Was Raw

I have already mentioned the phrase. Take the red pill. Wake up. Escape the matrix. But the red pill isn't just a metaphor from a film. It's a symbolized capsule of mammoth blood. The matrix? Your inflamed hippocampus. Wakefulness tastes like zinc-rich liver and frost-sharpened clarity.

It's the marrow our grandmothers sucked from bones when the fields lay barren. It's the copper-tang of liver on your tongue beneath a hunter's moon, not the chalk dust of pills in a fluorescent-lit pharmacy. It's hunger that teaches and fat that remembers. Truth isn't swallowed. It's bled. You've swallowed truth in muscle and marrow. And truth doesn't digest. It becomes you.

This isn't politics. This isn't self-help. This is ancestral memory reactivated in flesh. And the people who fear it? They fear not your plate, but your clarity. Because you can now see what they've trained themselves not to see: That the world is sick, and it likes it that way.

You Are Not the Same

Look back. Think of who you were before this began. You were told to eat small. To snack constantly. To fear cholesterol. To distrust your hunger. To count, to log, to obey.

You were told that fruit was good, and fat was evil. That soy was smart, and steak was violence. That weakness was empathy and discipline was oppression.

But you saw through it. You chose steak over status. Fasting over fear. Sunlight over screen light. Stillness over stimulation. Meat over media. Blood over branding.

And now, your breath is slower. Your gaze is stronger. Your cravings no longer own you. Your silence unsettles people who used to outrank you. This wasn't a bio hack. It was a return to form. You are not 'healed.' You are awake. And if you need proof? It's in your blood. Your new physiology:

- **Dawn cortisol peak**: 18–22 µg/dL (not flattened)
- **Postprandial ketones**: 1.5–3.0 mM (metabolic flexibility)
- **hs-CRP**: <0.5 mg/L (inflammation silenced)

These numbers aren't goals. They're ancestral birthrights reclaimed.

I Am the Vampire. And So Are You.

Yes. It's time I said it clearly. I am the vampire. The one who walked through famine and empire, through firelight and fluorescent lies, and remembered. I chose hunger over sedation. Meat over myth. Fire over fear. I chose to stay behind, not to rule, but to ignite. I am not immortal. I am ancestral. Not undying. Just unforgotten.

And you? You have become what I am. Not cursed, chosen. Not parasitic, prophetic. Your fangs aren't for necks. They're for tearing lies from their roots. And they're growing... 0.3mm a year, say the marrow-fed anthropologists[1].

Your thirst isn't for blood. It's for the silence before dawn, when the world forgets to lie. That silence tastes of iron and frost and needs no prescription. You do not fear death. You fear forgetting.

That is what makes you one of us now. Not your diet. Your devotion. Not your macros. Your memory. Not you just existing. You are living... and really living.

You Are the Red Flame Now

So, what now? Now that you've remembered. You go back into the world. Not to argue. Not to convert. To burn. Let them mock your meals. Let them whisper about your fasts. Let them laugh at your fat and fear your clarity. They will call you extreme. They will call you dangerous. They will call you mad. Smile. Because you know. They are starving. And you have fed.

Now live like flame. Eat like a god. Fast like a mystic. Rest like a lion. Move like a shadow. Speak only when your hunger is true. Let them clutch their smoothies and mutter about moderation. You know the truth now: Moderation is a leash.

Remember, the Spartans starved their boys to teach hunger's wisdom. Then feasted them on melas zomos - black broth of blood, vinegar, and the courage of boars who faced spears. Melas zomos wasn't just broth. It was liquid courage, drunk from skull-cups under wolf-starred skies. Modern 'moderation' would've died at first sip[2].

Let your LDL cholesterol preach louder than their pills. Let your ketones hymn the heresy of hunger. Let your strength be your sermon. Raise your children with meat and memory. Let your bloodline remember. Be the one who breaks the generational fog. The one who hunts. The one who heals. The one who reclaims the feast.

The Journey Never Ends - It Returns.

This was never about reaching the end. There is no finish line. There is only the flame, handed down, carried forward, burning brighter each time it's remembered.

You've walked with me this far. But now I step back. Because you are not behind me. You are beside me. And ahead of me. I am not your master. I am your memory. You are the fire now. You are the one who walks. You are the one who waits. You are the one who remembers.

And when others are ready, when their hunger becomes more than physical. You will not lecture. You will not market. You will burn. They will feel it. They will remember. And they will follow the flame.

Eat like your ancestors are watching and smiling. Speak with the certainty of a body that's reclaimed its birthright. Let your plate be your protest. Let your silence cut deeper than swords. The epilogue isn't an ending. It's your first hunt as the flame.

Epilogue

The Fire That Walks

A Gospel of Remembrance

Author's Preface

This is not a fable. Not entertainment. Not even story. This is memory, buried in myth, waiting to burn. It is a tale I once lived. And so did you.

Some truths cannot be taught directly. They must be remembered sideways, through hunger, through silence, through story.

You've made it this far. You've fasted, feasted, and awakened. Now, read this not as fiction. Read it as recognition.

Time is not a line. Time is a flame. And some fires walk.

A Tale from Before Time Remembered

They said the world began with light. They were wrong. The world began with hunger. Long before cities or calendars, before the gods had names.

There lived a tribe whose bones were carved from mountain and whose blood sang the songs of stars. They hunted not to eat, but to remember. To forget the hunger was to forget who you were.

In this tribe was a boy, small, strong-eyed, and strange. He did not laugh when others laughed. Did not sleep when others slept. He fasted long past the feasting days. He stood too still when elders spoke of spirits. And sometimes, they said, he stared through people, as if watching something behind their eyes.

His name was Toma: those who wait. A name not given by chance, but by time itself.

One winter, the cold came early and would not leave. Game vanished. Mothers whispered. Children cried for warmth.

And on the third night of the hunger moon, Toma vanished into the woods with nothing but a flint knife and a strip of dried meat, meat he did not eat. They thought him dead. Or possessed. Or both.

But what returned on the seventh night was not the boy. It wore his shape, but the shape moved differently. It did not blink as much. It did not shiver. And its eyes, those eyes were lit from within, as though a coal smoldered behind them, refusing to die.

His footsteps left no snow-crunch, only the smell of iron and frost. When he breathed, the air did not mist. He bore no kill. No firewood. No wounds. Only a phrase, repeated like a prayer: "The fire walks."

The tribe spoke of Them, beings neither alive nor dead, who hunted in silence, fed in shadow, and knew the true names of stars. They called them ghosts, demons… gods.

Toma knew better. They were what we used to be. They came to him now, not in dreams, but in remembrance. He fasted, and they spoke. He stood beneath the moon, and they approached, not with footsteps, but with presence. And when he followed them, into the caves, the dark groves, the places even wolves avoided, he was not afraid. Because they did not harm him.

They taught him. How to move without sound. How to eat without shame. How to wait without wasting. How to kill cleanly and bless the blood. But most of all, they taught him not to forget.

One night, in the third year of the long hunger, Toma followed a figure he had seen only in flicker and fire, tall, cloaked, neither old nor young, skin like cooled ash over embers, voice like bone striking bone.

The figure never turned. Never looked back. But it knew Toma. Knew his steps. Knew his breath. Knew the question pulsing in him like a second heart: Why me?

They climbed for hours in silence. Higher than the wind dared go. Into a cave blacker than blindness. And there, at the mouth of the world, the figure spoke, not in words, but in truth: "You were not chosen. You were remembered."

And in that moment, the water pierced him like shards of night, and in that shattering, he saw: Mountains rising and crumbling like bread crusts. Tribes hunting, forgetting, hunting again. His own face, older, younger, always staring back from every reflection in every age. He saw the world as it truly was, not a line, but a spiral. Not progress, but pattern. A burning ring. A blood-soaked wheel. A cycle of hunger and fire and forgetting. He saw himself not as a boy, but as a return. A recurrence. A revenant.

This path was no stranger to his feet. He had walked it not once, not twice, but through lifetimes. And the figure beside him? He had taught him before. And been taught by him. For time was not a line. It was a flame. And the fire walked.

They say the gods live above the sky. But that is not true. The gods live in the bone. And the only way to reach them is to be hollowed first.

The figure did not name himself, and Toma did not ask. Names belonged to the living. And this, this was older than names. Their days were not measured in sunrises, but in stillness, fasting, and repetition.

For seven days, Toma ate nothing. Not as punishment, but as preparation. "You cannot be filled until you are hollow," the firewalker said. "The body forgets truth when it is full of lies. You must hunger to remember."

At first, Toma's limbs trembled. Then they steadied. His thoughts, once noisy, became sharp and silent. The fear drained. The noise of the world fell away like smoke.

And when, at last, he stood in the cold wind beneath a sky blackened with stars, his body became something else, not just stronger, but clearer. A blade. A flame. A vessel for something old.

The rites began. They hunted with bare hands, not for the kill, but for the rite. The firewalker taught him to track not footprints, but patterns in silence. To smell the cold before it arrived. To hear the heartbeat of prey across the wind.

Their first kill was a lean-blooded stag. They did not cut its throat. They whispered to it. And when it stopped moving, when it surrendered, Toma saw it clearly: It was not prey. It was an offering. A memory in fur and muscle.

They ate at night. In silence. Flesh first. Fat last. Liver always. No berries. No roots. No leaf. The firewalker growled softly when Toma asked why. "Plants survive by forgetting. Plants beg you to forget, they grow thorns and poisons. Meat remembers. Meat invites remembrance. When you eat the stag, you swallow its courage. When you eat the boar, you inherit its defiance. The liver is where the animal's fire burned brightest, eat it to reclaim yours."

Toma grew lean. Then sharp. Then still. His hunger became joy. His body burned, not from cold, but from something within. A warmth not fed by fire, but by return.

And then came the final rite. "The body does not lie," the firewalker said. "The lie is that you were ever anything but this. Time must crack to let the fire through."

He led Toma to a frozen pool beneath the mountain's peak. There was no reflection. Only constellations, burning where his face should be.

And Toma stepped into the water, though it burned colder than bone. A silent thunder cracked through his marrow. And in that instant... he saw. He was not just Toma. He was the firewalker. He had taught these rites before. He had died. Returned. Forgotten. Remembered. The fire had always walked in him. He was the one who waits, because he had waited through centuries, for himself.

The figure turned to him now, no longer taller. No longer stranger. They were the same. One in flesh. One in memory. Two ends of the flame. The firewalker placed a hand on his chest. "You are now the one who walks. I may vanish. But you, you burn."

Toma descended the mountain in silence. The snow did not crunch beneath his feet. The wind parted for him. He did not shiver. He carried no weapon. No torch. Only the fire inside.

When he returned to the tribe, the children hid. The elders bowed, not in fear, but in something older … recognition. No one asked where he had gone. Some truths are too sacred for questions.

But the world had changed in his absence. The hunger moon had stretched into a hunger year. Berries were bitter. Roots turned black. The fleshless were dying. And still, no one hunted.

Toma watched them gnaw bark and pray to sky gods that never answered. Watched them dig into dirt, searching for sustenance in shadows. Watched them feed their children fear disguised as wisdom. He did not scold. He did not shout. He simply waited.

And when one young boy, a mirror of himself, asked: "Why don't you eat like us?" Toma smiled with a warmth that came from bone and blood. "Because I remember."

That night, he built no fire. He roasted no meat. He sat cross-legged in the dark and let the scent of his strength speak for him. They came, one by one, not with questions, but with silence. A stillness settled over them, deeper than the night cold, as if the air itself held its breath.

A mother touched Toma's arm and jerked back as if scalded. "You're hot," she whispered. He smiled. "No. You've been cold too long." They felt it. The truth is not taught. It is transmitted. There was no test. No sermon. Only silence, and the words he carried: "You've forgotten who you are. But I came back to remind you."

Seasons turned. The tribe changed. They began to fast, not in punishment, but in praise. They remembered how to hunt, not for sport, but for memory. They began to eat in silence, until the meat touched the tongue. Then they sang.

Liver was sacred. Fat was holy. Blood was remembrance. And when a child asked, "Where is Toma now?" The elders pointed to their own chests. "Here. And here. And here."

For the fire walks in all who refuse to forget. And the name they once feared, The Fire That Walks, became a blessing passed from elder to child: "Walk like the fire. Feed like the flame. Speak only when your hunger is true." But all things burn. Even memory.

One day, Toma walked into the woods and did not return. Some said he died. Others said he turned into mist. The elders knew better. He had become the flame.

You thought it was just a tale. But you've met the firewalker before. In the hunger-cave of your cravings, on the third day of your own fast. In the silence between meals. In the first cut of meat that reminded your cells who they are.

He was not a stranger. He was your shadow. Your future. Your past. Your reflection. You were not changed. You were revealed. This was not entertainment. This was initiation. 'The fire that walks' is not a metaphor. It is a truth remembered in flesh. It moves through those who awaken. It hunts in silence. It burns in blood. And now, because your blood burns, it walks in you.

Burn so bright, they'll mistake you for the sun,
while their world starves in the shadows
of their own moderation.

References

Chapter 1: Myths We've Been Fed

1. Ravnskov, U. The Cholesterol Myths. New Trends Publishing, 2000.
2. Teicholz, N. The Big Fat Surprise. Simon & Schuster, 2014.
3. Hite, A.H., et al. "In the face of contradictory evidence…" Nutrition, 2010.
4. Szalai, J. "John Harvey Kellogg and the Cereal Crusade." The New York Times Review of Books, 2017.
5. Shanahan, C. Deep Nutrition. Flatiron Books, 2017.
6. Nestle, M. Food Politics: How the Food Industry Influences Nutrition and Health. University of California Press, 2002.
7. Gundry, S.R. The Plant Paradox. Harper Wave, 2017.
8. Fung, J. The Obesity Code. Greystone Books, 2016.
9. Eswaran, S., et al. "Fiber and functional GI disorders." The American Journal of Gastroenterology, 2013.
10. Turnbaugh, P.J., et al. "The human microbiome project." Nature, 2007.
11. Park, Y., et al. "Dietary fiber intake and risk of colorectal cancer." JAMA, 2005.
12. Holick, M.F. "Vitamin D deficiency." The New England Journal of Medicine, 2007.
13. Wacker, M., & Holick, M.F. "Sunlight and vitamin D." Dermato-Endocrinology, 2013.
14. Palacios, C., & Gonzalez, L. "Is vitamin D deficiency a major global public health problem?" J Steroid Biochem Mol Biol, 2014.
15. Bikle, D.D. "Vitamin D metabolism, mechanism of action, and clinical applications." Chemistry and Biology, 2014.

16. Valtin, H. "'Drink at least eight glasses of water a day.' Really?" American Journal of Physiology, 2002.

17. Guyton, A.C., & Hall, J.E. Textbook of Medical Physiology, 12th ed. Saunders, 2011.

18. Siri-Tarino, P.W., et al. "Meta-analysis of saturated fat and coronary heart disease." Am J Clin Nutr, 2010.

19. Mozaffarian, D., et al. "Diet and long-term weight gain." The New England Journal of Medicine, 2011.

20. McDonough, A.A., et al. "Regulation of sodium balance and blood pressure by the kidney." Comprehensive Physiology, 2012.

21. Murray, R.K., et al. Harper's Illustrated Biochemistry, 30th ed. McGraw-Hill, 2015.

22. Gammage, L.C., et al. "Veganism and the environment: what are the consequences?" Environment, Development and Sustainability, 2021.

23. Martin, W.F., et al. "Dietary protein intake and renal function." Nutrition & Metabolism, 2005.

24. Veech, R.L. "The therapeutic implications of ketone bodies." Prostaglandins, Leukotrienes and Essential Fatty Acids, 2004.

25. Cahill, G.F. "Fuel metabolism in starvation." Annual Review of Nutrition, 2006.

26. Longo, V.D., & Panda, S. "Fasting, circadian rhythms, and time-restricted feeding." Cell Metabolism, 2016.

27. National Academies of Sciences. Dietary Reference Intakes: Macronutrients. National Academies Press, 2005.

Chapter 2: Dracula Doesn't Do Carbs

1. Longo, V.D. et al. (2014). Fasting: Molecular Mechanisms and Clinical Applications. Cell Metabolism, 19(2), 181–192.

2. Ahima, R.S. (2009). Ghrelin and hunger. NEJM, 360(9), 875–877.

3. Muller, T.D., et al. (2015). Ghrelin. Molecular Metabolism, 4(6), 437–460.

4. Cheng, C.W., et al. (2014). Prolonged fasting reduces IGF-1 and promotes hematopoietic stem cell regeneration. Cell Stem Cell, 14(6), 810–823.

5. Youm, Y.H., et al. (2015). Ketogenic diet reduces midlife mortality and improves memory in aging mice. Cell Metabolism, 22(3), 427–437.

6. Johnson, R.J., et al. (2007). Fructose in metabolic syndrome. Hypertension, 50(3), 613–619.

7. Uribarri, J., et al. (2010). AGEs in food and reduction strategies. JADA, 110(6), 911–916.

8. Ibid.

9. Newman, J.C., & Verdin, E. (2014). Ketone bodies as signaling metabolites. Trends Endocrinol Metab, 25(1), 42–52.

10. D'Agostino, D.P., et al. (2013). Therapeutic ketosis with ketone supplementation. Epilepsy Res, 100(3), 304–314.

11. Cunnane, S.C., et al. (2016). Brain energy rescue for neurodegeneration. Nat Rev Drug Discov, 15(7), 492–503.

12. Poff, A.M., et al. (2014). Ketone supplementation decreases tumor cell viability. Front Nutr, 1, 10.

13. Hultkrantz, Å. (1987). The vision quest. JAAR, 55(1), 35–47.

14. Brown, J.E. (1953). The sacred pipe: Black Elk's account of the seven rites of the Oglala Sioux.

15. Schultes, R.E., et al. (2019). Fasting and vision states in Sioux Sundance. J Ethnopharmacol, 233, 20–27.

16. Tinsley, G.M., et al. (2016). Time-restricted feeding and resistance training. Eur J Sport Sci, 16(7), 843–852.

17. Manoogian, E.N.C., & Panda, S. (2017). Circadian feeding and healthy aging. Ageing Res Rev, 39, 59–67.

18. Longo, V.D., & Panda, S. (2016). Fasting and lifespan. Cell Metab, 23(6), 1048–1059.

19. Brand, M.D. (2000). Mitochondrial inefficiency in ageing. Exp Gerontol, 35(6–7), 811–820.
20. Meydani, S.N., et al. (2004). Caloric restriction and immunity. J Gerontol, 59(7), 697–700.
21. Yilmaz, Ö.H., et al. (2012). Diet and stem cell regulation. Cell Stem Cell, 10(6), 502–511.
22. Jung, C.G. (1951). Aion: Phenomenology of the Self.
23. Longo, V.D., et al. (2021). Fasting: Molecular Mechanisms. Cell Metab, 33(11), 2111–2126.
24. D'Agostino, D.P., et al. (2013). Ketone-induced GABA modulation. Epilepsy Res, 100(3), 304–314.
25. Mattson, M.P., et al. (2017). Intermittent metabolic switching. Ageing Res Rev, 39, 46–58.
26. Paoli, A., et al. (2015). Ketogenic diet and phytonutrients. JISSN, 12(1), 1–7.
27. Cahill, G.F. (2006). Fuel metabolism in starvation. Annu Rev Nutr, 26, 1–22.
28. Randle, P.J., et al. (1963). The glucose fatty-acid cycle. The Lancet, 281(7285), 785–789.

Chapter 3: The Turning

1. Cahill, G. F. (2006). Fuel metabolism in starvation. Annual Review of Nutrition, 26, 1–22.
2. Phinney, S. D., & Volek, J. S. (2011). The Art and Science of Low Carbohydrate Living. Beyond Obesity LLC.
3. Noakes, T. D. (2008). Waterlogged: The Serious Problem of Overhydration in Endurance Sports. Human Kinetics.
4. Sonnenburg, J. L., & Sonnenburg, E. D. (2015). The Good Gut: Taking Control of Your Weight, Your Mood, and Your Long-term Health. Penguin.
5. DiNicolantonio, J. J., & O'Keefe, J. H. (2020). The Salt Fix: Why the Experts Got It All Wrong - and How Eating More Might Save Your Life. Harmony.

6. Belkaid, Y., & Hand, T. W. (2014). Role of the microbiota in immunity and inflammation. Cell, 157(1), 121–141.

7. de Groot, P. F., et al. (2017). Gut microbiota composition in obesity and metabolic dysfunction. Scientific Reports, 7(1), 1–13.

8. Vasan, K., et al. (2020). Beta-hydroxybutyrate as a signaling metabolite. Trends in Endocrinology & Metabolism, 31(4), 297–309.

9. Weber, D. D., et al. (2021). Ketogenic diets and mitochondrial function: An updated review. International Journal of Molecular Sciences, 22(2), 989.

10. Kovatcheva-Datchary, P., et al. (2015). Diet modulates gut microbiota and improves glucose tolerance in humans. Cell Metabolism, 22(6), 971–982.

11. Evrensel, A., & Ceylan, M. E. (2015). The gut-brain axis: The missing link in depression. Clinical Psychopharmacology and Neuroscience, 13(3), 239–244.

12. Sayin, S. I., et al. (2013). Gut microbiota regulates bile acid metabolism by reducing the levels of tauro-beta-muricholic acid, a naturally occurring FXR antagonist. Cell Metabolism, 17(2), 225–235.

Chapter 4: You Are Not Cattle

1. Lustig, R. H. (2013). Fat Chance. Penguin.

2. Trut, L., Oskina, I., & Kharlamova, A. (2009). BioEssays, 31(3), 349–360.

3. Hare, B., & Tomasello, M. (2005). Trends in Cognitive Sciences, 9(9), 439–444.

4. Larsen, C. S. (2006). Quaternary International, 150(1), 12–20.

5. Cordain, L., et al. (2005). Am J Clin Nutr, 81(2), 341–354.

6. Armelagos, G. J. (2014). In Human Diet and Nutrition.

7. Stefansson, V. (1956). Not by Bread Alone. Macmillan.

8. Mann, G. V. (1964). J Atherosclerosis Res, 4, 289–312.

9. Kaplan, H. et al. (2017). The Lancet, 389(10080), 1730–1739.

10. Scott, J. C. (2017). Against the Grain. Yale University Press.

11. Taubes, G. (2008). Good Calories, Bad Calories. Vintage.

12. Ziker, J. P. (2002). Peoples of the Tundra. Waveland Press.

13. Vitebsky, P. (2005). The Reindeer People. Houghton Mifflin Harcourt.

14. Norwitz, N. G., et al. (2021). Front Psychiatry, 12, 1–18.

Chapter 5: The Original Diet Was Red

1. Domínguez-Rodrigo, M. et al. (2005). "Cutmarks on bone surfaces and their implications for reconstructing early hominin behavior." Journal of Human Evolution, 48(1), 109–121.

2. Aiello, L. C., & Wheeler, P. (1995). "The Expensive-Tissue Hypothesis." Current Anthropology, 36(2), 199–221.

3. Wrangham, R. (2009). Catching Fire: How Cooking Made Us Human. Basic Books.

4. Bramble, D. M., & Lieberman, D. E. (2004). "Endurance running and the evolution of Homo." Nature, 432(7015), 345–352.

5. Beasley, D. E. et al. (2015). "The evolution of stomach acidity and its relevance to the human microbiome." PLOS ONE, 10(7), e0134116.

6. Larsen, C. S. (2006). "The agricultural revolution as environmental catastrophe: Implications for health and lifestyle in the Holocene." Quaternary International, 150(1), 12–20.

7. Cohen, M. N., & Armelagos, G. J. (1984). Paleopathology at the Origins of Agriculture. Academic Press.

Chapter 6: Blood, Brine, and Bone

1. Milton, K. (1999). A hypothesis to explain the role of meat-eating in human evolution. Evolutionary Anthropology, 8(1), 11–21.
2. National Institute of Diabetes and Digestive and Kidney Diseases. (2023). Your Digestive System & How it Works. https://www.niddk.nih.gov
3. Beasley, D. E., Koltz, A. M., Lambert, J. E., Fierer, N., & Dunn, R. R. (2015). The evolution of stomach acidity and its relevance to the human microbiome. Biology Letters, 11(4), 20150207. https://doi.org/10.1098/rsbl.2015.0207
4. Verhaegen, M., Munro, S., & Puech, P. F. (2002). Aquarboreal ancestors? Medical Hypotheses, 59(3), 308–313. https://doi.org/10.1016/S0306-9877(02)00204-6
5. Mann, N. (2000). Meat in the human diet: An anthropological perspective. Nutrition & Dietetics, 57(1), 19–26.
6. Wrangham, R. (2009). Catching Fire: How Cooking Made Us Human. Basic Books.
7. Ben-Dor, M., Barkai, R., & Sirtoli, R. (2021). The evolution of the human trophic level during the Pleistocene. American Journal of Physical Anthropology, 175(1), 3–16. https://doi.org/10.1002/ajpa.24247
8. Larsen, C. S. (2006). The Agricultural Revolution as Environmental Catastrophe: Implications for Health and Lifestyle in the Holocene. Quaternary International, 150(1), 12–20

Chapter 7: The Salt That Remembers

1. Leviticus 2:13, The Holy Bible.
2. Kurlansky, M. (2002). Salt: A World History. Vintage.
3. Volek, J.S., & Phinney, S.D. (2011). The Art and Science of Low Carbohydrate Living. Beyond Obesity LLC.

4. Noakes, T. (2012). Waterlogged: The Serious Problem of Overhydration in Endurance Sports. Human Kinetics.
5. Eaton, S.B., et al. (1997). "Evolutionary Health Promotion." Preventive Medicine, 27(5), 691–700.
6. Hall, J.E. (2015). Guyton and Hall Textbook of Medical Physiology (13th ed.). Elsevier.
7. Sebastian, A., et al. (2002). "Paleolithic Nutrition: Evidence from Modern Hunter-Gatherers." European Journal of Nutrition, 41(2), 61–70.
8. DiNicolantonio, J.J., & Lucan, S.C. (2014). "The Wrong White Crystals: Not Salt but Sugar as Aetiological in Hypertension and Cardiometabolic Disease." Open Heart, 1(1), e000167.
9. Graudal, N.A., et al. (2014). "Compared With Usual Sodium Intake, Low- and Excessive-Sodium Diets Are Associated With Increased Mortality." American Journal of Hypertension, 27(9), 1129–1137.
10. Frassetto, L.A., et al. (2000). "Diet, Evolution and Aging: The Pathophysiologic Effects of the Post-agricultural Inversion of the Potassium-to-Sodium Ratio." European Journal of Nutrition, 39(2), 67–70.

Chapter 8: The Undying Mind

1. de la Monte SM. (2008). Alzheimer's disease is type 3 diabetes. J Diabetes Sci Technol, 2(6), 1101–1113.
2. Mosconi L. (2005). Brain glucose metabolism in Alzheimer's disease. Eur J Nucl Med Mol Imaging, 32(4), 486–510.
3. Cunnane SC et al. (2011). Brain fuel metabolism in Alzheimer's disease. PNAS, 109(48), 19673–19678.
4. Courchesne-Loyer A et al. (2016). Ketones as an alternative brain fuel. Curr Opin Clin Nutr Metab Care, 19(6), 434–439.

5. Veech RL. (2004). The therapeutic implications of ketone bodies. Prostaglandins Leukot Essent Fatty Acids, 70(3), 309–319.

6. Youm YH et al. (2015). Ketone bodies inhibit NLRP3 inflammasome. Nat Med, 21(3), 263–269.

7. Cheng CW et al. (2014). FOXO3a and PGC-1α in lifespan extension. Science, 339(6116), 211–214.

8. Swanson RA et al. (2021). Amyloid-β pathology: 30 years of evolution. Nat Rev Neurol.

9. Zlokovic BV. (2008). Clearing amyloid from the brain. Rev Neurosci, 16(2), 99–111.

10. Mattson MP. (2016). BDNF and brain health. Cold Spring Harb Perspect Med, 6(7), a029843.

11. Sleiman SF et al. (2016). Ketones increase hippocampal BDNF. J Neurochem, 139(5), 769–781.

12. Harhaj NS, Antonetti DA. (2014). BBB integrity and ketones. Neuroscience, 278, 1–10.

13. Fortier M et al. (2020). Ketogenic drink in MCI. Neurobiol Aging, 86, 54–62.

14. Newport MT. (2013). What If There Was a Cure?

15. Taylor MK et al. (2021). Ketogenic therapy improves cognition. Clin Nutr, 40(9), 5045–5052.

16. Roberts SB et al. (2017). Skipping breakfast and cognitive performance. Am J Clin Nutr.

17. Taylor MK et al. (2018). Efficacy of MCTs in mild cognitive impairment. J Alzheimer's Dis.

Chapter 9: The Suntan Vampire

1. Zasada, M., Budzisz, E. (2019). Biological effects of retinoids on skin. Postepy Dermatol Alergol, 36(4), 392–397. https://doi.org/10.5114/ada.2019.91398

2. Ogawa, Y., Kinoshita, M., Shimada, S., Kawamura, T. (2018). Zinc and skin disorders. Nutrients, 10(9), 199. https://doi.org/10.3390/nu10091202

3. Veech, R. L. (2004). The therapeutic implications of ketone bodies: effects in pathological conditions. Prostaglandins, Leukotrienes and Essential Fatty Acids, 70(3), 309–319.

4. Feingold, K. R. (2007). The role of epidermal lipids in cutaneous permeability barrier homeostasis. J Lipid Res, 48(12), 2531–2546. https://doi.org/10.1194/jlr.R700013-JLR200

5. Chen, A. C.-H., Martin, A. J., Choy, B., et al. (2015). A Phase 3 Randomized Trial of Nicotinamide for Skin-Cancer Chemoprevention. NEJM, 373(17), 1618–1626. https://doi.org/10.1056/NEJMoa1506197

6. Pilkington, S. M., Watson, R. E., Nicolaou, A., & Rhodes, L. E. (2011). Omega-3 polyunsaturated fatty acids: photoprotective macronutrients. Exp Dermatol, 20(7), 537–543. https://doi.org/10.1111/j.1600-0625.2011.01289.x

7. Ramsden, C. E., et al. (2013). Dietary linoleic acid and its role in skin inflammation and UV damage. BMJ Open, 3(3), e002002. https://doi.org/10.1136/bmjopen-2012-002002

8. Larsen, C. S. (1995). Biological changes in human populations with agriculture. Ann Rev Anthropol, 24, 185–213. https://doi.org/10.1146/annurev.an.24.100195.001153

Chapter 10: The Fat Phobia Ritual

1. Astrup, A. et al. (2020). J Am Coll Cardiol, 76(7), 844–857.

2. Dobs, A.S. et al. (2012). Journal of Clinical Endocrinology, 97(4), 458–465.

3. Volek, J.S., & Phinney, S.D. (2011). The Art and Science of Low Carbohydrate Living.

4. Newman, J.C., & Verdin, E. (2014). Trends Endocrinol Metab, 25(1), 42–52.#
5. Krauss, R.M. (2006). Curr Opin Lipidol, 17(4), 393–398.
6. Ramsden, C.E. et al. (2013). BMJ, 346:e8707.
7. Teicholz, N. (2014). The Big Fat Surprise.
8. Santos, F.L. et al. (2020). Obesity Reviews, 21(7), e13045.
9. Astrup, A. et al. (2020). J Am Coll Cardiol, 76(7), 844–857.

Chapter 11: The Predator's Pantry

1. Bramble, D.M., & Lieberman, D.E. (2004). Endurance running and the evolution of Homo. Nature, 432(7015), 345–352.
2. Aiello, L.C., & Wheeler, P. (1995). The expensive-tissue hypothesis. Current Anthropology, 36(2), 199–221.
3. Wrangham, R., et al. (1999). The raw and the stolen: cooking and the ecology of human origins. Current Anthropology, 40(5), 567–594.
4. Outram, A.K. (2004). Food for thought: why did modern humans kill and eat mammoths? Archaeology International, 8(1), 22–25.
5. Lee, R.B. (1979). The !Kung San: Men, Women, and Work in a Foraging Society. Harvard University Press.
6. Liebenberg, L. (2006, 2008). Persistence hunting by modern hunter-gatherers. Current Anthropology, 47(6), 1017–1026.
7. Pontzer, H., et al. (2021). Evolutionary energetics and human biology. Annual Review of Anthropology, 50, 461–478.
8. Lombard, M., et al. (2021). Tracking cognition: The neural mechanisms of persistence hunting. Evolutionary Anthropology, 30(5), 236–247.

9. Cordain, L., et al. (2000). Plant-animal subsistence ratios and macronutrient energy estimations in worldwide hunter-gatherer diets. AJCN, 71(3), 682–692.
10. Lieberman, D.E. (2021). Hunt, Gather, Parent: What Ancient Cultures Can Teach Us About Raising Children. Chapter: "The Hunter's Brain", pp. 92–114.
11. Woodburn, J. (1982). Egalitarian societies. Man, 17(3), 431–451.
12. Gubser, N.J. (1965). The Nunamiut Eskimo. Yale University Press.

Chapter 12: Why Nature Never Served Protein Alone

1. Cunnane, S.C., et al. (2016). "Brain energy rescue: ketones supply energy to the aging brain." Neurobiology of Aging, 38, 27–34.
2. Barendregt, L. et al. (2022). "Mitochondrial dysfunction in high-protein, low-fat diets." Cell Metabolism, 34(4), 549–561.
3. Cahill, G.F. Jr. (2006). "Fuel metabolism in starvation." Annual Review of Nutrition, 26, 1–22.
4. Heinbecker, P. (1931). "Studies on the Metabolism of Eskimos." Journal of Biological Chemistry, 92(2), 615–622.
5. Watanabe, M., et al. (2004). "Cholesterol and sex hormone synthesis." Endocrine Reviews, 25(4), 535–538.
6. Shearer, M.J., & Newman, P. (2008). "Metabolism and cell biology of vitamin K." Thrombosis and Haemostasis, 100(4), 530–547.
7. Stefansson, V. (1913). My Life with the Eskimo. Macmillan.
8. Baulieu, E.E., et al. (2001). "Neurosteroids: of the nervous system, by the nervous system, for the nervous

system." Recent Progress in Hormone Research, 56, 329–357.

9. Stefansson, V. (1913). My Life with the Eskimo. Macmillan.

10. Cordain, L., et al. (2000). "Plant-animal subsistence ratios in hunter-gatherer diets." American Journal of Clinical Nutrition, 71(3), 682–692.

11. Mann, N. et al. (2012). "Hadza energy intake and macronutrient balance." American Journal of Clinical Nutrition, 95(6), 1603–1611.

12. Schaller, G.B. (1972). The Serengeti Lion: A Study of Predator-Prey Relations. University of Chicago Press.

13. Zeisel, S.H., et al. (2003). "Choline, egg yolks, and brain development." Nutrition Today, 38(2), 55–62.

14. Morton, R.W., et al. (2018). "A systematic review, meta-analysis and meta-regression of the effect of protein supplementation on resistance training–induced gains in muscle mass and strength in healthy adults." British Journal of Sports Medicine, 52(6), 376–384.

15. Teicholz, N. (2016). "The scientific report guiding the US dietary guidelines: is it scientific?" BMJ Evidence-Based Medicine, 21(2), 64–68.

Chapter 13: Sacred Blood, Forbidden Flesh

1. Detienne, M. & Vernant, J.-P. (1989). The Cuisine of Sacrifice Among the Greeks. University of Chicago Press.

2. Kahan, B. (2014). The Laws of Shechita. Feldheim Publishers.

3. The Torah, Leviticus 17:11 (JPS Tanakh).

4. Campo, J. E. (2009). Encyclopedia of Islam. Infobase Publishing.

5. Carrasco, D. (1999). City of Sacrifice: The Aztec Empire and the Role of Violence in Civilization. Beacon Press, p. 114.

6. Pelikan, J. (1985). Jesus Through the Centuries: His Place in the History of Culture. Yale University Press, ch. "The Cosmic Christ," pp. 196–202.

7. DeMallie, R.J. (Ed.). (2001). Handbook of North American Indians: Plains, Vol. 13. Smithsonian Institution, p. 896.

8. Beard, M. (1980). "The Sexual Status of Vestal Virgins." Journal of Roman Studies, 70, 12–27.

Chapter 14: The Nightshade and the Nightmare

1. Mensinga TT, Sips AJ, Rompelberg CJ, van Twillert K. (2005). A physiologically based toxicokinetic (PBTK) model for the potato glycoalkaloid α-solanine: toxic effects and human exposure. RIVM Report 340720003.

2. Patel S. (2018). Solanine toxicity thresholds: human safety estimates. Journal of Food Science, 83, T1–T7.

3. Fasano A. (2012). Leaky gut and autoimmune diseases. Clinical Reviews in Allergy & Immunology, 42(1), 71–78.

4. Genomics England. (2023). Frequency of HLA-B27 in UK populations. Genomics England Research Portal.

5. Holmes RP, Assimos DG. (2004). The impact of dietary oxalate on kidney stone formation. Urological Research, 32(5), 311–316.

6. Zimmermann MB. (2009). Iodine deficiency and goiter in the 21st century. Endocrine Reviews, 30(4), 376–408.

7. Monk JP et al. (2017). Oxalate content of modern spinach cultivars: impact of selective breeding. Journal of Agricultural and Food Chemistry, 65(14), 2842–2849.

8. Knight J et al. (2016). Oxalate nephropathy in patients consuming green smoothies. American Journal of Kidney Diseases, 68(1), 122–126.

Chapter 15: The Pulse of Death

1. Sathe, S.K. et al. (2018). "Bioactive compounds in legumes: Processing and bioavailability." Journal of Food Science, 83(1). PMID: 28915390.
2. van Vliet, S. et al. (2021). "Plant-Based Diets and Muscle Health." Nutrients, 13(1). PMID: 33253939.
3. Lopez, A. et al. (2017). "Micronutrients in human health." Critical Reviews in Food Science and Nutrition, 58(17). PMID: 28526025.
4. Postgate, J.N. (1992). Early Mesopotamia. Routledge.
5. Garnsey, P. (1999). Food and Society in Classical Antiquity. Cambridge University Press.
6. Davis, M. (2001). Late Victorian Holocausts. Verso.
7. Willett, W. et al. (2019). "Food in the Anthropocene." The Lancet, 393(10170), 447–492.
8. FAO. (2021). The State of Food Security and Nutrition in the World. Rome: FAO.
9. Levine, H. et al. (2017). "Temporal trends in sperm count." Human Reproduction Update, 23(6), 646–659.
10. See: Loucks, A.B. (2007). "Low energy availability in the marathon and other endurance sports." Clinical Journal of Sport Medicine, 17(5), 417–424.

Chapter 16: The Eternal Meal

1. Safrai, S. (1987). The Jewish People in the First Century. Van Gorcum.
2. Campo, J.E. (2009). Encyclopedia of Islam. Infobase Publishing.
3. Marlowe, F.W. (2010). The Hadza: Hunter-Gatherers of Tanzania. University of California Press.
4. Cummings, D.E. et al. (2001). A preprandial rise in plasma ghrelin levels suggests a role in meal initiation. Nature Neuroscience, 4, 229–233.

5. Panda, S. (2016). The Circadian Code, pp. 112–115.
    Rodale.
6. Mizushima, N. & Komatsu, M. (2011). Autophagy:
    Renovation of Cells and Tissues. Cell, 147(4), 728–741.
7. Cahill, G.F. Jr. (2006). Fuel Metabolism in Starvation.
    Annual Review of Nutrition, 26, 1–22.
8. Hartman, M.L. et al. (1992). Augmented growth hormone
    secretory burst frequency and amplitude during a two-day
    fast in normal men. Journal of Clinical Endocrinology &
    Metabolism, 74(4), 757–765.
9. Ho, K.Y. et al. (1988). Fasting Enhances Growth
    Hormone Secretion and Amplifies the Complex Rhythms
    of GH Secretion. The Journal of Clinical Investigation,
    81(4), 968–975.
10. Mattson, M.P. (2014). Fasting: Molecular Mechanisms and
    Clinical Applications. Nature Reviews Immunology, 14,
    760–774.
11. Volek, J.S. et al. (2006). Testosterone responses to
    intermittent fasting. Journal of Clinical Endocrinology &
    Metabolism, 91(9), 3453–3459.

Chapter 17: The Mirror of Meat

1. Miller, W.L. (2005). Minireview: Steroidogenic enzyme
    expression in the human fetal adrenal: physiology and
    pathology. Endocrinology, 146(7), 2645–2651.
2. Coad, J., & Conlon, C. (2021). Iron deficiency in women:
    assessment, causes and consequences. Current Opinion in
    Clinical Nutrition and Metabolic Care, 24(6), 440–445.
3. Smith, A.D. et al. (2018). Homocysteine, B vitamins, and
    cognitive impairment. Neurology, 91(18), e1711–e1721.
4. Price, W.A. (1939). Nutrition and Physical Degeneration.
5. Knapen, M.H.J. et al. (2015). Three-year low-dose
    menaquinone-7 supplementation helps decrease bone loss

in healthy postmenopausal women. Osteoporosis International, 26, 2499–2507.

6. Fernstrom, J.D. (2013). Large neutral amino acids: dietary effects on brain neurochemistry and function. Amino Acids, 45(3), 419–430.

7. Lynch, H. et al. (2018). Plant-Based Diets and Nutrient Deficiency in Female Athletes. Journal of the International Society of Sports Nutrition, 15, 43.

8. Chavarro, J.E. et al. (2008). Diet and lifestyle in the prevention of ovulatory disorder infertility. Obstetrics & Gynecology, 111(5), 1146–1153.

9. Klement, R.J. (2019). Beneficial Effects of Ketogenic Diets for Cancer Patients: A Realist Review. Nutrition, 67–68, 110548.

10. Hughes, C.L. et al. (2020). Soy Isoflavones and Reproductive Health: Mechanistic Insights. Journal of the Endocrine Society, 4(9), bvaa090.

11. Stefansson, V. (1956). Not By Bread Alone. Hill and Wang. (See p.78 for cardiovascular comparisons in Inuit populations.)

12. Bègue, L. et al. (2022). Red meat and aggression: Investigating stereotypes with empirical analysis. Psychological Science, 33(9), 1458–1470.

13. Hsieh, M.H. et al. (2020). Association Between Dietary Patterns and Amenorrhea in Women. Journal of Clinical Endocrinology & Metabolism, 105(11), dgaa487.

14. Fontana, F. et al. (2021). Diet and Male Testosterone Levels: Effects of Plant-Based Patterns. Molecular Nutrition & Food Research, 65(10), 2000721.

Chapter 18: The Cold-Blooded Ritual

1. Janssen, L. G., et al. (2022). Cold-induced norepinephrine increases in humans. iScience, 25(3), 105009.

2. Hanssen, M. J., et al. (2022). Cold exposure and lipolysis: synergistic effects with fasting. Diabetes, 71(10), 2112–2123.

3. Takahashi, H., et al. (2021). FGF21 is a cold-induced hepatokine that enhances ketogenesis via PGC-1α signaling. Nature Metabolism, 3(2), 219–229.

4. Zhang, Y., et al. (2023). Combined fasting and cold exposure enhance hippocampal BDNF and neurogenesis. Cell Reports, 42(1), 110001.

5. Iwen, K. A., et al. (2018). Cold-induced brown adipose tissue activity in healthy adults. Journal of Clinical Endocrinology & Metabolism, 103(9), 3389–3399.

6. Chevalier, C., et al. (2020). Cold shock proteins as regulators of inflammation. EMBO Journal, 39(15), e104068.

7. Boutant, M., et al. (2017). Cold exposure activates PGC-1α-dependent mitochondrial biogenesis in skeletal muscle. Cell Metabolism, 25(5), 1009–1026.

8. Cannon, B., & Nedergaard, J. (2004). Brown adipose tissue: function and physiological significance. Physiological Reviews, 84(1), 277–359.

9. Andersen, K. L. (1960). Cold acclimatization and shivering thresholds in Arctic populations. Journal of Applied Physiology, 15(4), 637–640.

10. Stefansson, V. (1956). Not by Bread Alone. Macmillan.

11. Rodahl, K. (1949). Vitamin A content and toxicity of bear and seal liver. Journal of the American Medical Association, 139(5), 370–373.

Chapter 19: The Blood of the Child

1. CDC. (2020). Prevalence of Prediabetes Among Adolescents and Young Adults. MMWR, 69(2), 97–103.

2. CDC. (2022). Dietary Guidelines for Added Sugars in Children.

3. Nestel, P. et al. (1989). Hemoglobin concentrations in East African pastoralists. American Journal of Clinical Nutrition, 49(1), 62–70.

4. Stefansson, V. (1956). Not By Bread Alone. Hill and Wang.

5. Marlowe, F.W. (2010). The Hadza: Hunter-Gatherers of Tanzania. University of California Press.

6. Cartledge, P. (2003). The Spartans: An Epic History. Vintage.

7. Livy. (c. 27 BC). Ab Urbe Condita.

8. Sommerburg, O. et al. (2015). Retinol vs. Beta-Carotene Absorption in Children. Journal of Nutrition, 145(5), 1142S–1148S.

9. Haskell, M. et al. (2005). Bioefficacy of beta-carotene in children. American Journal of Clinical Nutrition, 82(4), 795–803.

10. Wang, D.D. et al. (2022). Linoleic acid-rich oils in US school lunches. Nutrition Reviews, 80(3), 324–336.

11. Ouellet, V. et al. (2011). BAT activation in humans during cold exposure. Journal of Clinical Endocrinology & Metabolism, 96(1), 63–69.

12. Schleicher, R.L. et al. (2016). Vitamin D intake and status in US children. American Journal of Clinical Nutrition, 104(3), 619–627.

13. Cultural Survival. (2013). The Dukha: Last Reindeer Herders of Mongolia.

14. Baatjargal, B. et al. (2017). Urban vs. rural asthma in Mongolian children. European Respiratory Journal, 50(Suppl 61), PA1102.

15. Miller, J.D. et al. (2019). Vitamin D status in Mongolian herder children. Public Health Nutrition, 22(7), 1317–1324.

Chapter 20: The Fire That Doesn't Bleed

1. Cunnane, S. (2020). Ketones: The fourth fuel. Annual Review of Nutrition.
2. Goss, A. M. (2020). Ketogenic diet for menopausal symptoms. Menopause, 27(5), 584–592.
3. DeSouza, M. J. (2021). Protein needs in menopause. Current Opinion in Clinical Nutrition.
4. Koutnik, A. P. (2023). Effects of a carnivore diet on insulin resistance in menopausal women. Journal of Nutritional Biochemistry, 115, 108989.
5. Lambert, M. A. (2022). Reduction in hot flashes with animal-based ketogenic nutrition. Maturitas, 162, 29–34.
6. Ventura-Clapier, R. (2017). Estrogen modulation of mitochondrial fusion and bioenergetics. Molecular Metabolism, 6(6), 678–692.
7. Demarest, T. G. (2022). Menopause and mitophagy in neural and metabolic systems. Nature Aging, 2(1), 1–10.
8. Stachenfeld, N. S. (2022). Sodium restriction increases cortisol in postmenopausal women. American Journal of Physiology: Endocrinology and Metabolism.
9. Laskowski, D. A. (2021). High-meat diets improve bone density in postmenopausal women. Journal of Bone and Mineral Research, 36(11), 2091–2103.
10. Bacon, B. R. (2020). Heme iron intake and genetic risk of iron overload. Blood, 136(Supplement 1), 26.

Chapter 21: The Misfit's Hunger

1. Frye, R. E., et al. (2013). Mitochondrial dysfunction in autism spectrum disorders. Frontiers in Pediatrics, 1, 22.
2. Cervenka, M. C., et al. (2017). The ketogenic diet for epilepsy and beyond. JAMA Neurology, 74(5), 500–506.

3. Gál, E. M., et al. (2022). Metabolic and nutritional strategies in ADHD: a review. Nutritional Neuroscience, 25(8), 1624–1634.

4. Cunnane, S. C., et al. (2020). Ketones as brain fuel in aging and neurodegenerative disease. Clinical Nutrition, 39(4), 1146–1152.

5. Ramsden, C. E., et al. (2012). Linoleic acid and the risk of neurodegeneration. Prostaglandins, Leukotrienes and Essential Fatty Acids, 87(1), 35–41.

6. Yeagle, P. L. (1989). Cholesterol and the cell membrane. Biochimica et Biophysica Acta, 1008(2), 231–234.

7. Dean, C., & Keshavan, M. (2017). The role of cholesterol in synapse formation and plasticity. Translational Psychiatry, 7(1), e1019.

8. Palmer, C. M. (2022). Brain Energy: A Revolutionary Breakthrough in Understanding Mental Health. BenBella Books.

9. Pulsifer, M. B., et al. (2001). Ketogenic diet in treatment of ADHD: preliminary data. Journal of Child Neurology, 16(9), 722–723.

10. Kirkpatrick, C. F., et al. (2020). Nutritional interventions for ADHD: A systematic review. Nutrients, 12(6), 1596.

11. Hedger, N., et al. (2021). Visual threat detection in autism: Faster but different. Autism Research, 14(2), 312–321.

12. Hagen, E. H., et al. (2020). Cognitive performance and foraging behavior in ADHD. Evolution and Human Behavior, 41(3), 219–229.

13. Chang, J. C., et al. (2023). Serum cholesterol and neural conduction in ADHD. JAMA Psychiatry, 80(2), 102–110.

14. Volkow, N. D., et al. (2017). Saturated fat intake and dopamine signaling in the reward system. Molecular Psychiatry, 22(8), 1230–1236.

15. Kitson, C. N., et al. (2023). Oxidized linoleic acid metabolites and anxiety in mice. Journal of Lipid Research, 64(2), 200–212.

16. Rose, S., et al. (2021). Mitochondrial fragmentation in autism and response to ketogenic therapy. Cell Reports, 36(5), 109612.
17. Horder, J., et al. (2018). Glutamate and GABA imbalance in autism. Neuropsychopharmacology, 43(2), 240–248.
18. Knight, R. E., et al. (2021). Oxalate toxicity and neural deposition in sensory pathways. Neurology Reviews, 29(4), 183–190.

Chapter 22: The Vampire's Code

1. Sato, M., et al. (2014). Chronobiology International, 31(10), 1101–1110.
2. Poggiogalle, E., et al. (2018). Journal of Endocrinology, 238(2), R185–R205.
3. LeGates, T. A., et al. (2014). Nature Reviews Neuroscience, 15(8), 470–481.
4. Repacek, A. D., et al. (2022). PNAS, 119(21), e2120453119.
5. Medic, G., et al. (2017). Nature and Science of Sleep, 9, 151–161.
6. Cote, K. A., et al. (2023). Journal of Clinical Endocrinology & Metabolism, 108(1), 72–79.
7. Chaix, A., et al. (2019). Cell Metabolism, 29(3), 591–604.
8. Kalam, H., et al. (2023). Cell Reports Medicine, 4(8), 101141.
9. Schoenfeld, B. J., et al. (2015). Nutrition Reviews, 73(2), 69–82.
10. Vieira, A. F., et al. (2021). Journal of Applied Physiology, 130(4), 1041–1050.
11. McAllister, M., et al. (2023). JAMA Psychiatry, 80(2), 134–142.
12. Mizushima, N., & Komatsu, M. (2011). Cell, 147(4), 728–741.
13. Xie, L., et al. (2013). Science, 342(6156), 373–377.

14. Mestre, H., et al. (2020). Science, 367(6475), 528–531.
15. Longo, V. D., & Panda, S. (2016). Cell Metabolism, 23(6), 1048–1059.
16. Heinonen, I. H., et al. (2022). Frontiers in Physiology, 13, 836320.
17. Volkow, N. D., et al. (2017). Nature Reviews Neuroscience, 18(12), 741–752.
18. Tinsley, G. M., & La Bounty, P. M. (2015). JISSN, 12(1), 4.
19. Yamaguchi, T., et al. (2018). Complementary Therapies in Medicine, 40, 117–123.
20. Lopez, R., et al. (2023). Journal of Digital Psychology, 5(1), 33–42.
21. Martel, J., et al. (2020). Journal of Immunology Research, 2020, 2562054.

Chapter 23: Organs and Ancestors

1. Warren, J. M., et al. (2021). "Nutrient composition of organ meats." Journal of Food Composition.
2. Anderson, K. (2023). "Comparative bioavailability of animal-sourced vitamin A." Journal of Nutritional Biochemistry.
3. Obeid, R., et al. (2005). "Folate and vitamin B12 status in meat-eaters, vegetarians and vegans." Clinical Chemistry and Laboratory Medicine.
4. Chang, J., et al. (2022). "Brain phospholipids and neurogenesis." Scientific Reports.
5. UK FSA (2021). "BSE risk assessment and ruminant offal." Food Standards Agency Bulletin.
6. Tavassoli, M., et al. (2021). "Marrow adipocytes and MSC precursors." Stem Cells.
7. Morris, R., et al. (2022). "Steroidogenic content of bovine testes." Journal of Animal Science.

8. Tihonen, K., et al. (2020). "Prayer-induced vagal tone and digestion." American Journal of Physiology.
9. Dunn, C., et al. (2023). "Neurogastronomic reverence and micronutrient uptake." Behavioral Nutrition Review.
10. Petrovic, L., et al. (2023). "PFAS and toxin accumulation in CAFO vs. pasture organs." Environmental Health Perspectives.
11. Peterson, A., et al. (2022). "Aflatoxin bioaccumulation in confined cattle." Toxicology in Agriculture.
12. Gahan, M., et al. (2021). "Exosomal inheritance and transgenerational memory." Epigenetics and Chromatin.
13. European Commission (2023). "Directive on freezing protocols for raw meat." CELEX:32023R0123.

Chapter 24: The Heart That Hides

1. Barber, P. (1988). Vampires, Burial, and Death: Folklore and Reality. Yale University Press.
2. Weatherford, J. (2004). Genghis Khan and the Making of the Modern World. Crown.
3. Hite, A. et al. (2023). "Oxidative Stress Markers in Nomadic vs. Agrarian Graves." Scientific Reports, 13(1).
4. DiNicolantonio, J., & O'Keefe, J.H. (2018). "The Importance of Dietary Cholesterol." Open Heart, 5(1), e000785.
5. Zampelas, A. et al. (2022). "LDL-C and Cognitive Function in the Elderly." Neurology, 98(15), 1640–1648.
6. Kraft, D. et al. (2020). "Postprandial Glucose and Retinal Response." Investigative Ophthalmology & Visual Science, 61(14), 28.
7. Becker, E. (1973). The Denial of Death. Free Press.
8. Austrian Military Report on Peter Plogojowitz (1725).
9. Seyfried, T. (2015). Cancer as a Metabolic Disease. Wiley.
10. Capriles, E. (2004). The Dzogchen Teachings. Snow Lion.

11. Lipson, E. (2010). "The Rainbow Body Phenomenon." Journal of Consciousness Studies, 17(9–10), 204–232.
12. Cheng, Z. et al. (2021). "Fasting-Induced Chaperone-Mediated Autophagy in Monastic Communities." Cell Metabolism, 33(4), 748–765.

Chapter 25: The Infected Herd

1. Gregory, J. et al. (2023). HbA1c and COVID-19 Mortality: A Nationwide Study of 1.2 Million Patients. The Lancet Diabetes & Endocrinology, 11(3), 141–150.
2. Codo, A. et al. (2020). Elevated glucose levels favor SARS-CoV-2 infection and monocyte response. Cell Metabolism, 32(3), 437–446.e5.
3. Kroemer, G. et al. (2024). Hyperglycemia amplifies viral replication in human airway tissue. Cell, 187(1), 112–125.e8.
4. Bikman, B. (2020). Why We Get Sick. BenBella Books.
5. Malhotra, A. (2022). A Statin-Free Life. Yellow Kite.
6. Nauck, M.A. et al. (2023). HbA1c and COVID-19 Risk Stratification. JAMA, 329(2), 141–153.
7. Goldberg, A. et al. (2023). Ketones Suppress NLRP3 Inflammasome to Mitigate Cytokine Storm. Science Immunology, 8(16), eadh0186.
8. Nørgaard, M. et al. (2023). Linoleic Acid Induces Hyperinflammation in Viral Infection. Immunity, 59(4), 715–729.
9. Read, T. et al. (2024). Zinc Lozenges Reduce Viral Shedding Duration: A Randomized Controlled Trial. JAMA Network Open, 7(4), e245670.
10. Charoenngam, N. et al. (2023). Vitamin D and COVID-19 Outcomes: A Meta-analysis. Nutrients, 15(2), 449.
11. Anderson, H. et al. (2023). Nutrient Density of Beef Liver vs. Plant Sources. Journal of Ancestral Health, 4(1), 33–44.

12. Cheng, Y. et al. (2024). Fasting Induces Naïve T-Cell Proliferation and Immune Renewal. Nature Immunology, 25(2), 223–234.
13. Gurven, M. et al. (2021). Sickness Behavior and Recovery in Tsimane Foragers. American Journal of Human Biology, 33(5), e23520.

Chapter 26: The Hollowing

1. Müller, T. D., et al. (2022). GLP-1 and the regulation of appetite and food intake. Nature Metabolism.
2. Khan, M. A., et al. (2021). Effects of GLP-1 agonists on bone metabolism. Journal of Clinical Endocrinology & Metabolism.
3. Riggs, B. L., et al. (2023). Accelerated bone loss in GLP-1 treated women. Journal of Bone and Mineral Research.
4. Schwartz, A. V., et al. (2016). Loss of lean body mass with GLP-1 receptor agonists. The Lancet Diabetes & Endocrinology.
5. Tan, T. M., et al. (2017). Gastrointestinal side effects of GLP-1-based therapies. Obesity Reviews.
6. Kravitz, H. M., et al. (2022). GLP-1 drugs and reproductive axis disruption. Endocrine Reviews.
7. Wild, R. A., et al. (2023). Amenorrhea associated with GLP-1 analogues: case series and review. Fertility and Sterility.
8. Terhune, C., & Respaut, R. (2023). Maker of Wegovy, Ozempic showers money on U.S. obesity doctors. Reuters Investigates.
9. BBC News. (2024). Wegovy pricing disparity draws scrutiny. BBC.
10. European Medicines Agency. (2024). Safety review of GLP-1 receptor agonists. EMA Public Statement.
11. Patel, S. A., et al. (2024). Facial fat pad changes in GLP-1 drug users. Plastic and Reconstructive Surgery.

12. Goss, A. M., et al. (2021). Iron repletion restores ovulation in iron-deficient women. Journal of Clinical Endocrinology & Metabolism.

Chapter 27: Gut Healing & Immune Reset

1. Fasano, A. (2012). "Zonulin and its regulation of intestinal barrier function." Physiological Reviews.
2. Erridge, C. (2010). "Endotoxin and the gut-liver axis in health and disease." The American Journal of Physiology.
3. Carrera-Bastos, P. et al. (2011). "The Western diet and lifestyle and diseases of civilization." Research Reports in Clinical Cardiology.
4. Schnorr, S. L. et al. (2014). "Gut microbiome of the Hadza hunter-gatherers." Nature Communications.
5. Louis, P. et al. (2014). "Short chain fatty acids and human colonic function." Current Opinion in Clinical Nutrition and Metabolic Care.
6. Kovacs-Nolan, J. et al. (2005). "Egg yolk antibodies (IgY) for passive immunity." Annual Review of Food Science and Technology.
7. Sannasiddappa, T. H. et al. (2017). "Bile acids disrupt biofilms formed by Enterococcus faecalis." Scientific Reports.
8. Wahlström, A. et al. (2016). "Bile acids in regulation of metabolism." The Journal of Lipid Research.
9. Sonnenburg, J. L. & Bäckhed, F. (2016). "Diet–microbiota interactions." Nature.
10. Gershon, M. D. (1998). The Second Brain. HarperCollins.
11. Cryan, J. F. et al. (2019). "The microbiota–gut–brain axis." Nature Reviews Neuroscience.
12. Yano, J. M. et al. (2015). "Indigenous bacteria regulate host serotonin." Cell.
13. Blunt, J. (2020). Personal interview, BBC Radio 4.

14. Levine, M. et al. (1996). "Vitamin C pharmacokinetics." Proceedings of the National Academy of Sciences.
15. Ghosh, S. et al. (2020). "High-fat diets and intestinal barrier function." Current Opinion in Clinical Nutrition and Metabolic Care.
16. Chevalier, G. et al. (2012). "Earthing: Health implications of reconnecting the human body to the Earth's surface electrons." Journal of Environmental and Public Health.
17. Food Standards Agency (2020). "Raw liver: safety and freezing guidelines." UK Government Food Hygiene Advice.

Chapter 28: The Cell That Forgot

1. Liberti MV, Locasale JW. Trends Biochem Sci. 2016;41(3):211–218.
2. Warburg O. Nobel Laureates Conference, Lindau, Germany, 1966.
3. Seyfried TN. Cancer as a Metabolic Disease. Wiley; 2012.
4. Vasan N, et al. Nature. 2023;615(7950):329–334.
5. Seyfried TN. Front Oncol. 2023;13:1175812.
6. Mizushima N, Komatsu M. Cell. 2011;147(4):728–741.
7. Newman JC, Verdin E. Annu Rev Nutr. 2017;37:51–76.
8. Seyfried TN, D'Agostino DP. Front Oncol. 2020;10:628.
9. Klement RJ. Cancers. 2020;12(9):2379.
10. Weber DD, Aminzadeh-Gohari S, et al. J Clin Oncol. 2022;40(16_suppl):2012.
11. Weber DD, Aminzadeh-Gohari S, et al. Clin Nutr. 2018;37(6):2060–2067.
12. Di Biase S, Longo VD, et al. Cell. 2017;168(5):775–789.e12.
13. de Groot S, et al. Cell. 2020;181(5):1096–1112.e18.

Chapter 29: The Undrugged Mind

1. Nowak, C. et al. (2023). Statin-induced new-onset diabetes in normoglycemic individuals. JAMA Intern Med, 183(1), 44–55.

2. Hidaka, T. et al. (2022). Rosuvastatin-associated CoQ10 depletion and cardiac diastolic dysfunction. ESC Heart Failure, 9(3), 1887–1896.

3. Ott, D. et al. (2024). Long-term statin use and hippocampal atrophy. Neurology, 102(5), e209121.

4. Ravnskov, U. et al. (2016). LDL-C Does Not Cause Cardiovascular Disease. Expert Rev Clin Pharmacol, 9(10), 1337–1346.

5. Mach, F. et al. (2020). LDL and innate immunity. Atherosclerosis, 311, 1–9.

6. Kruth, H.S. et al. (2023). LDL as an immune LPS binder. Nature Immunol, 24(1), 11–18.

7. Domanski, M. et al. (2017). Oxidized LDL and cardiovascular risk. Curr Atheroscler Rep, 19(3), 21.

8. Mason, P. et al. (2024). Seed oil peroxides glycate LDL 8x faster than glucose. J Lipid Res, 65(2), 109–121.

9. Jonsson, T. et al. (2018). Cardiovascular health in Iceland pre-statin era. Scand J Public Health, 46(2), 163–170.

10. Maalouf, M., Rho, J.M., & Mattson, M.P. (2009). Neuroprotective properties of ketone bodies. Brain Res Rev, 59(2), 293–315.

11. Kashiwaya, Y. et al. (2023). Ketone-induced mitochondrial proliferation in neurons. Cell Metab, 35(4), 677–692.

Chapter 30: The Bloodline

1. Brillat-Savarin, J.A. (1825). Physiologie du Goût. Paris: Sautelet.

2. Banting, W. (1863). Letter on Corpulence, Addressed to the Public. London.

3. The Lancet. (1864). "Corpulence and Its Quacks." The Lancet, 83(2122), 525–526.

4. Stefansson, V. (1929). Adventures in Diet. Harper's Monthly, Nov.

5. JAMA. (1929). "The Bellevue Experiment: A Reckless Diet." JAMA, 93(3), 214.

6. Carpenter, K.J. (1986). "The History of Scurvy and Vitamin C." Cambridge University Press.

7. Ebstein, W. (1882). Zur Therapie der Fettleibigkeit. Wiesbaden: J.F. Bergmann.

8. Ebstein, W. (1883). "Fettdiät und Gicht." Berliner Klinische Wochenschrift, 20(17), 345–350.

9. Deutsches Ärzteblatt. (1902). "Gegen die Fett-Diät." May 12, p. 843.

10. Allen, F.M. (1919). Total Dietary Regulation in the Treatment of Diabetes. Rockefeller Institute.

11. Allen, F.M. (1921). "Prolonged Diabetic Survival Without Insulin." Journal of Metabolic Research, 2(4), 287–294.

12. Petrén, K. (1923). "Behandlung des Diabetes mit fettreicher Kost." Svenska Läkarsällskapets Handlingar, 49, 112–118.

13. Lutz, W. (1967). Leben ohne Brot. Gießen: Aurelia Verlag.

14. Yudkin, J. (1972). Pure, White and Deadly. London: Davis-Poynter.

15. Kearns, C.E., Schmidt, L.A., & Glantz, S.A. (2016). "Sugar Industry and Coronary Heart Disease Research." JAMA Internal Medicine, 176(11), 1680–1685.

16. Wellcome Library Archives (2024). "Yudkin Manuscript on Sugar and Liver Lipogenesis."

17. Kwaśniewski, J. (1999). Optimal Nutrition. Warsaw: WGP.

18. European Commission. (1998). Report on Unconventional Dietary Practices. SANCO/1394/98.

19. Bernstein, R.K. (1997). Dr. Bernstein's Diabetes Solution. Boston: Little, Brown.
20. American Diabetes Association. (1989). "Standards of Medical Care." Diabetes Care, 12(Suppl 1).
21. Bernstein, R.K. (1991). Personal Archive. https://www.diabetes-book.com.
22. TIME Magazine. (1963). "The Safflower Swindle." TIME, August 16, p. 41.

Chapter 31: The Red Flame

1. J. Anthropol. Res. (2023). Marrow-Rich Diets and Odontometric Adaptation: Longitudinal Analysis of Canine Growth in Ketogenic Populations.
2. Plutarch, Lycurgus, 12.3: "Melas zomos - black broth of vinegar and blood - formed the sacred feast of Spartan endurance. Drunk not in comfort, but ceremony."

www.ingramcontent.com/pod-product-compliance
Lightning Source LLC
Chambersburg PA
CBHW051712020426
42333CB00014B/954